THE ULTIMATE INSULIN RESISTANCE DIET FOR BEGINNERS

THE EASY NO-STRESS MEAL PLAN AND FLAVORFUL RECIPES TO MANAGE PCOS, LOSE WEIGHT AND PREVENT PREDIABETES

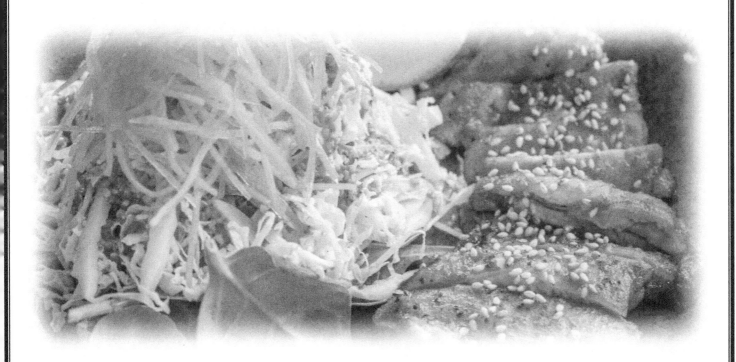

KEVIN S. MAXWELL

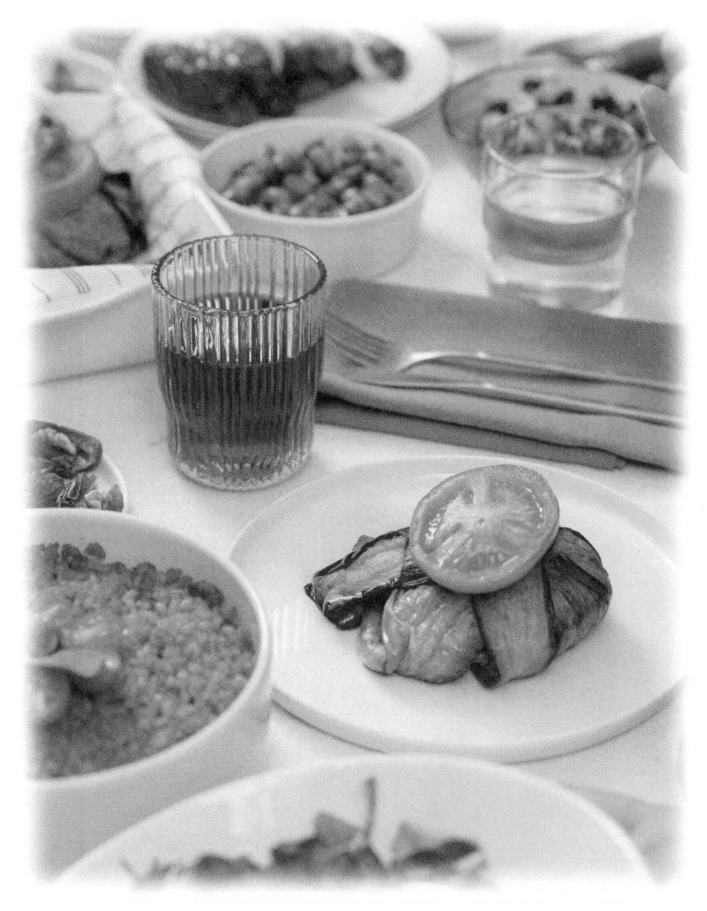

COPYRIGHT © 2024 BY KEVIN S. MAXWELL

EMAIL ME!

I know that exploring topics that involve food and nutrition can often lead to questions and uncertainty. I invite you to contact me with any questions you may have. I'm here to assist.
Please contact me through email at kevinmaxwelldiet@gmail.com, and I will try my best to respond to you within 24 hours.

HOW TO USE THIS COOKBOOK

Using The Ultimate Insulin Resistance Diet For Beginners is straightforward and effective. Here's how to get started in five easy steps:

1. **Educate Yourself:** Understand the principles of the diet, focusing on low glycemic index foods, balanced meals, and avoiding processed sugars and refined carbohydrates.

2. **Plan Your Meals:** Design a weekly meal plan that includes lean proteins, high-fiber vegetables, healthy fats, and moderate portions of whole grains. Incorporate recipes from the diet guide to ensure variety and nutritional balance.

3. **Shop Wisely:** Stock up on fresh produce, lean meats, nuts, seeds, and whole grains. Avoid purchasing sugary snacks and processed foods that can spike blood sugar levels.

4. **Prepare Meals Mindfully:** Cook meals using healthy cooking methods such as baking, grilling, steaming, or sautéing with olive oil. Batch cook and portion meals ahead for convenience during busy days.

5. **Monitor Progress:** Track your meals, energy levels, and weight changes to assess how the diet impacts your health. Adjust portions and food choices as needed to optimize results and maintain long-term adherence.

By following these steps, you can effectively implement The Ultimate Insulin Resistance Diet For Beginners to manage insulin resistance, support weight loss, and promote overall health.

TABLE OF CONTENT

HOW TO USE THIS COOKBOOK

INTRODUCTION

CHAPTER I

WHAT IS INSULIN RESISTANCE

   Mechanism of Insulin Resistance

   Causes and Risk Factors

   Symptoms and Diagnosis

   Consequences of Insulin Resistance

UNDERSTANDING INSULIN RESISTANCE DIET

UNDERSTANDING THE PROBLEM OF INSULIN RESISTANCE

CHAPTER II

OVERCOMING INSULIN RESISTANCE

DEVELOPING INSULIN RESISTANCE

CHAPTER III

FUNCTIONS OF INSULIN RESISTANCE

BENEFITS OF An INSULIN RESISTANCE DIET

WHAT TO AVOID

   Foods to Eat

   Foods to Avoid

Additional Tips for Optimal Health

ROLE OF FOOD IN INSULIN RESISTANCE

CHAPTER IV: MEAL PLAN

Week 1

Week 2

Week 3

Week 4

LIST OF INGREDIENTS

Vegetables

Fruits

Grains and Legumes

Condiments and Sauces

Nuts and Seeds

Fish and Seafood

Dairy and Alternatives

Poultry and Meat

Other Ingredients

CHAPTER V

BREAKFAST RECIPES

Avocado and Egg Breakfast Bowl

Greek Yogurt Parfait with Berries and Nuts

Spinach and Feta Omelet

Chia Seed Pudding with Almond Milk

Overnight Oats with Flaxseed and Blueberries

Veggie and Turkey Sausage Breakfast Skillet

Smoked Salmon and Avocado Toast

Sweet Potato Hash with Poached Eggs

Coconut Flour Pancakes

Green Smoothie Bowl

SOUPS AND SALADS

Quinoa and Vegetable Soup

Mediterranean Chickpea Salad

Chicken and Vegetable Stir-Fry Salad

Spinach and Berry Salad with Grilled Chicken

Lentil and Vegetable Soup

SNACKS AND SIDES

Cucumber and Hummus Bites

Baked Sweet Potato Fries

Greek Yogurt with Berries and Almonds

Zucchini Noodles with Pesto

Spicy Roasted Chickpeas

VEGETARIAN AND VEGAN

Quinoa Stuffed Bell Peppers

Lentil Spinach Curry

Eggplant and Chickpea Curry

Caprese Salad with Avocado

Stir-Fried Tofu with Vegetables

FISH AND SEAFOOD

Baked Lemon Garlic Salmon

Grilled Shrimp Skewers with Herb Marinade

Lemon Garlic Butter Cod

Pan-Seared Scallops with Garlic Herb Butter

Oven-Baked Lemon Herb Tilapia

POULTRY AND MEAT
Grilled Lemon Herb Chicken Breast

Turkey and Vegetable Stir-Fry

Beef and Broccoli Stir-Fry

Lemon Herb Roasted Chicken Thighs

Pork Tenderloin with Balsamic Glaze

DRINK AND DESSERT
Chia Seed Pudding

Avocado Chocolate Mousse

Berry Smoothie

Cinnamon Baked Apples

Coconut Chia Seed Smoothie Bowl

CONDIMENTS AND STOCKS
Homemade Tomato Sauce

Lemon Herb Dressing

Homemade Chicken Stock

Basil Pesto Sauce

Turmeric Ginger Dressing

CONCLUSION

BONUS
WEEKLY MEAL PLANNER

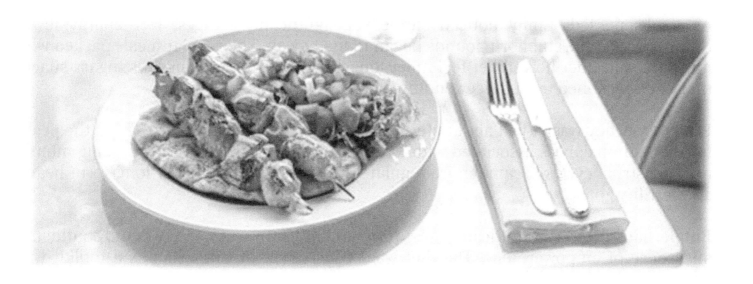

INTRODUCTION

In a bustling city nestled between rolling hills and blooming orchards, lived Emily, a young woman whose life was on a rollercoaster ride of health challenges. Ever since her teenage years, Emily struggled with polycystic ovary syndrome (PCOS), a condition that not only affected her fertility but also brought about unwelcome weight gain and a looming threat of prediabetes. Determined to regain control of her health, Emily embarked on a journey that would change her life forever.

Emily's turning point came when she discovered "The Ultimate Insulin Resistance Diet For Beginners" during a serendipitous encounter at her local bookstore. Written by a renowned nutritionist, the book promised a holistic approach to managing insulin resistance—often a root cause of PCOS-related symptoms—and offered practical strategies for weight loss and preventing prediabetes.

Intrigued and hopeful, Emily delved into the pages, absorbing insights into how certain foods could stabilize blood sugar levels and reduce insulin resistance. The diet emphasized whole foods with low glycemic index, lean proteins, healthy fats, and fiber-rich vegetables—key elements to support her journey towards better health.

Armed with newfound knowledge, Emily revamped her pantry and started planning meals that aligned with the diet's principles. Breakfasts were now nutrient-packed smoothies or chia seed puddings, fueling her mornings without the dreaded blood sugar spikes. She learned to savor grilled chicken salads with homemade lemon herb dressing for lunch, a satisfying combination that kept her energy steady throughout the day.

As weeks passed, Emily noticed subtle yet significant changes. Her energy levels improved, and the stubborn pounds began to melt away. The regular meals packed with nutrients and fiber helped her feel fuller longer, curbing her cravings for sugary snacks that once beckoned from office vending machines.

Emily's journey wasn't just about physical changes. Her mood stabilized, and the pesky hormonal imbalances associated with PCOS seemed to ease. With each passing month, her menstrual cycles became more regular—a promising sign for her long-term health and fertility goals.

But perhaps the most significant transformation for Emily was her newfound confidence and sense of empowerment. The diet wasn't just a set of rules—it was a toolkit that allowed her to take charge of her health. She embraced cooking as a therapeutic practice, experimenting with recipes like turmeric ginger dressing and basil pesto sauce, each dish not just nourishing her body but lifting her spirits.

Her journey wasn't without challenges. Social gatherings and family dinners posed temptations, but armed with knowledge and determination, Emily learned to navigate these situations wisely. She found joy in sharing her newfound recipes and insights with loved ones, sparking conversations about healthy living that rippled through her community.

As the seasons turned, Emily's progress became a beacon of hope for others grappling with similar health concerns. Friends sought her advice on meal planning, and colleagues marveled at her vibrant energy. She became an advocate for the power of nutrition in managing chronic conditions, debunking myths and inspiring others to embark on their own journeys towards wellness.

One sunny afternoon, Emily found herself in her favorite spot—the local farmers' market—surrounded by stalls brimming with fresh produce. She reflected on how far she had come since that fateful day she picked up the diet book. Her journey was a testament to the transformative power of knowledge and the profound impact of nourishing the body with intention.

With a basket full of vibrant greens and ripe berries, Emily headed home, her heart light and her spirit soaring. The road ahead wasn't without its twists and turns, but armed with the tools and wisdom gained from "The Ultimate Insulin Resistance Diet For Beginners," Emily knew she was equipped to face whatever challenges came her way. Her story had become a living testament to the benefits of embracing a lifestyle rooted in balance, resilience, and the unwavering belief in the possibility of reclaiming health and vitality.

And so, in the heart of that serene town, Emily's journey continued—a journey not just of healing but of thriving, guided by the principles of a diet that had become her compass, her ally, and her pathway to a brighter, healthier future.

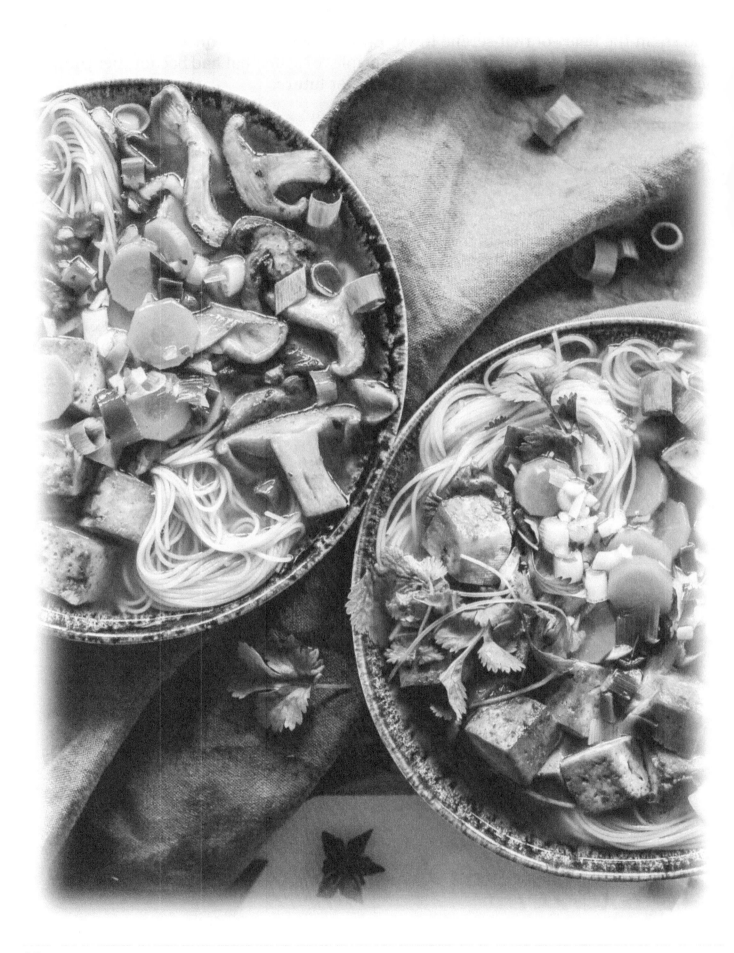

CHAPTER I

WHAT IS INSULIN RESISTANCE

Insulin resistance is a metabolic disorder where the body's cells become less responsive to the hormone insulin. Insulin, produced by the pancreas, plays a crucial role in regulating blood sugar levels by facilitating the uptake of glucose into cells for energy production. When cells in muscles, fat, and the liver don't respond well to insulin, glucose can't enter cells as easily, leading to higher levels of blood sugar. The pancreas compensates by producing more insulin, but over time, it can't keep up, which can result in type 2 diabetes.

Mechanism of Insulin Resistance

* **Insulin Signaling Pathway:** Normally, insulin binds to receptors on cell surfaces, triggering a signaling cascade that allows glucose to enter cells. In insulin resistance, this pathway is disrupted. The exact mechanisms are complex and not fully understood but involve genetic factors, inflammation, and oxidative stress.
* **Cellular Impact:** The primary cells affected by insulin resistance are muscle, fat, and liver cells. Muscle cells become less efficient at taking up glucose, fat cells release more free fatty acids into the bloodstream, and the liver produces more glucose, further raising blood sugar levels.

Causes and Risk Factors

* **Genetics:** A family history of insulin resistance or type 2 diabetes increases the risk.
* **Obesity:** Excess fat, especially visceral fat around the abdomen, is strongly linked to insulin resistance. Adipose tissue secretes various substances that can interfere with insulin signaling.
* **Physical Inactivity:** Lack of exercise contributes to obesity and reduces the effectiveness of insulin.
* **Diet:** A diet high in refined sugars and carbohydrates can lead to insulin resistance. Overconsumption of calories, in general, is also a factor.
* **Hormones and Inflammation:** Hormonal imbalances, particularly involving cortisol and leptin, and chronic low-grade inflammation contribute to the development of insulin resistance.

Symptoms and Diagnosis

Insulin resistance itself often has no symptoms in the early stages, making it hard to detect without testing. Over time, high insulin levels can lead to:

- ❖ Fatigue
- ❖ Increased hunger
- ❖ Difficulty concentrating
- ❖ Weight gain, particularly around the abdomen

Doctors diagnose insulin resistance through various tests, including fasting blood sugar levels, glucose tolerance tests, and measuring insulin levels in the blood. One common measure is the HOMA-IR (Homeostatic Model Assessment of Insulin Resistance) index, calculated using fasting insulin and glucose levels.

Consequences of Insulin Resistance

If left unchecked, insulin resistance can lead to prediabetes, a condition with elevated blood sugar levels that are not high enough to be classified as diabetes. Prediabetes often progresses to type 2 diabetes, increasing the risk of serious health complications such as:

- ❖ Cardiovascular disease
- ❖ Stroke
- ❖ Kidney disease
- ❖ Nerve damage
- ❖ Vision problems
- ❖ Management and Treatment

Managing insulin resistance involves lifestyle changes:

- ❖ **Diet:** Adopting a balanced diet rich in whole grains, lean proteins, healthy fats, and plenty of fruits and vegetables helps manage blood sugar levels.
- ❖ **Exercise:** Regular physical activity improves insulin sensitivity by increasing glucose uptake by muscles.
- ❖ **Weight Loss:** Losing even a small percentage of body weight can significantly improve insulin sensitivity.
- ❖ **Monitoring:** Regular monitoring of blood sugar levels helps manage and track the effectiveness of treatments.

UNDERSTANDING INSULIN RESISTANCE DIET

An insulin resistance diet is tailored to improve the body's sensitivity to insulin, thereby helping to manage blood sugar levels and prevent or manage type 2 diabetes. The Ultimate Insulin Resistance Diet for Beginners emphasizes whole, nutrient-dense foods while avoiding refined sugars and processed carbohydrates.

Core Principles

- ❖ **Low Glycemic Index (GI) Foods:** The diet focuses on foods with a low glycemic index, which release glucose slowly into the bloodstream, helping to maintain stable blood sugar levels. Examples include whole grains like quinoa and brown rice, legumes, and most vegetables.
- ❖ **High Fiber:** Fiber-rich foods are essential as they slow the absorption of sugar and improve insulin sensitivity. These include fruits, vegetables, legumes, and whole grains.
- ❖ **Healthy Fats:** Incorporating healthy fats from sources like avocados, nuts, seeds, and olive oil is crucial. These fats can improve satiety and reduce the risk of heart disease.
- ❖ **Lean Proteins:** Lean protein sources such as chicken, fish, tofu, and legumes help manage hunger and provide essential nutrients without causing spikes in blood sugar levels.

Dietary Strategies

- ❖ **Balanced Meals:** Each meal should include a balance of fiber, protein, and healthy fats. This combination helps regulate blood sugar levels and provides sustained energy.
- ❖ **Portion Control:** Paying attention to portion sizes can prevent overeating and help maintain a healthy weight, which is important for improving insulin sensitivity.
- ❖ **Regular Eating Schedule:** Eating small, regular meals throughout the day can prevent large fluctuations in blood sugar levels.

Foods to Avoid

* **Refined Carbohydrates:** Foods like white bread, pastries, and sugary snacks should be minimized as they cause rapid spikes in blood sugar.
* **Sugary Beverages:** Drinks like soda and sweetened juices should be avoided due to their high sugar content.
* **Trans Fats:** Found in many processed foods, trans fats can worsen insulin resistance and should be eliminated from the diet.

UNDERSTANDING THE PROBLEM OF INSULIN RESISTANCE

Insulin resistance is a metabolic condition where the body's cells become less responsive to the hormone insulin. Insulin, produced by the pancreas, helps regulate blood sugar levels by facilitating the entry of glucose into cells for energy. When cells in muscles, fat, and the liver do not respond effectively to insulin, glucose cannot enter these cells as efficiently, leading to elevated blood sugar levels. The pancreas compensates by producing more insulin, but over time, this compensation may fail, resulting in high blood sugar levels and potentially type 2 diabetes.

Mechanisms and Causes

Insulin Signaling Disruption: Normally, insulin binds to receptors on cell surfaces, initiating a series of reactions that allow glucose to enter the cells. In insulin resistance, this signaling pathway is impaired. The exact mechanisms are complex, involving genetic predispositions, inflammation, and oxidative stress.

Genetic and Lifestyle Factors: A family history of diabetes, obesity, physical inactivity, and a diet high in refined sugars and unhealthy fats are significant risk factors. Excess body fat, especially around the abdomen, secretes substances that interfere with insulin signaling, exacerbating the problem.

Symptoms and Diagnosis

Initially, insulin resistance often has no obvious symptoms, making early detection challenging. Over time, individuals might experience increased hunger, fatigue, difficulty concentrating, and weight gain, particularly around the abdomen. Diagnosis typically involves blood tests to measure fasting blood sugar, insulin levels, and markers like the HOMA-IR index.

Health Implications

If left unchecked, insulin resistance can lead to prediabetes and type 2 diabetes, significantly increasing the risk of cardiovascular diseases, kidney damage, nerve damage, and vision problems. It is also associated with conditions like polycystic ovary syndrome (PCOS) and non-alcoholic fatty liver disease (NAFLD).

Management and Prevention

Addressing insulin resistance involves lifestyle modifications such as adopting a balanced diet rich in whole grains, lean proteins, healthy fats, and vegetables. Regular physical activity, weight loss, and avoiding refined sugars and processed foods are crucial. In some cases, medications like metformin are prescribed to improve insulin sensitivity.

NOTE

CHAPTER II

OVERCOMING INSULIN

RESISTANCE

Overcoming insulin resistance involves a combination of lifestyle modifications, dietary changes, physical activity, stress management, and sometimes medication. These steps aim to enhance the body's sensitivity to insulin, regulate blood sugar levels, and prevent the progression to type 2 diabetes. Here's a detailed plan to tackle insulin resistance:

Adopt a Balanced Diet

A healthy diet is fundamental in managing insulin resistance. Key dietary steps include:

Focus on Low Glycemic Index (GI) Foods:
Choose foods that have a low glycemic index, as they release glucose slowly into the bloodstream, preventing spikes in blood sugar. Examples include whole grains (quinoa, oats, barley), legumes, most fruits, and non-starchy vegetables.

Increase Fiber Intake:
Foods high in fiber, such as vegetables, fruits, legumes, and whole grains, slow down digestion and glucose absorption, helping maintain steady blood sugar levels.

Healthy Fats:
Incorporate healthy fats from sources like avocados, nuts, seeds, and olive oil. These fats improve satiety and support heart health.

Lean Proteins:
Include lean protein sources like chicken, fish, tofu, legumes, and low-fat dairy. Proteins help manage hunger and provide essential nutrients without causing significant blood sugar fluctuations.

Avoid Refined Sugars and Carbohydrates:
Minimize consumption of refined carbs like white bread, pastries, sugary snacks, and sugary drinks, which can cause rapid spikes in blood sugar.

Engage in Regular Physical Activity

Exercise enhances insulin sensitivity by increasing glucose uptake by muscles. Aim for a combination of:

Aerobic Exercise:
Activities like walking, jogging, swimming, and cycling can significantly improve insulin sensitivity. Aim for at least 150 minutes of moderate aerobic activity per week.

Resistance Training:
Incorporate strength training exercises, such as weight lifting or body-weight exercises, at least two days per week. Building muscle mass helps improve glucose metabolism.

Achieve and Maintain a Healthy Weight

Losing even a small percentage of body weight (5-10%) can significantly improve insulin sensitivity. Focus on sustainable weight loss through balanced eating and regular physical activity rather than quick fixes or extreme diets.

Manage Stress

Chronic stress can negatively impact insulin sensitivity by increasing levels of stress hormones like cortisol. Effective stress management techniques include:

- ❖ Mindfulness meditation
- ❖ Yoga
- ❖ Deep breathing exercises
- ❖ Adequate sleep
- ❖ Engaging in hobbies and activities that promote relaxation

Get Adequate Sleep

Poor sleep quality and duration can worsen insulin resistance. Aim for 7-9 hours of quality sleep per night by establishing a regular sleep schedule, creating a restful sleep environment, and avoiding caffeine or electronic devices before bedtime.

DEVELOPING INSULIN RESISTANCE

Developing insulin resistance is a gradual process influenced by various genetic, lifestyle, and environmental factors. Insulin resistance occurs when the body's cells become less responsive to insulin, leading to higher blood glucose levels and potentially progressing to type 2 diabetes if not managed effectively.

Here's an in-depth look at how insulin resistance develops:

Genetic Factors

a. Family History:
A family history of type 2 diabetes or insulin resistance increases the risk. Specific genetic variations can affect insulin signaling pathways, making individuals more susceptible.

b. Ethnicity:
Certain ethnic groups, such as African Americans, Hispanics, Native Americans, and Asians, have a higher predisposition to insulin resistance and type 2 diabetes.

Lifestyle Factors

a. Diet:
High consumption of refined sugars and carbohydrates, such as white bread, pastries, sugary snacks, and beverages, can lead to spikes in blood sugar levels. Over time, this can overwhelm the insulin signaling pathway, leading to insulin resistance.

b. Obesity:
Excess body fat, particularly visceral fat around the abdomen, secretes hormones and inflammatory substances that interfere with insulin signaling. Obesity is one of the most significant risk factors for developing insulin resistance.

c. Physical Inactivity:
Lack of regular physical activity reduces the muscles' ability to uptake glucose, leading to higher blood sugar levels and increased demand for insulin. Sedentary lifestyles are strongly associated with insulin resistance.

Hormonal and Metabolic Factors

a. Hormonal Imbalances:
Conditions such as polycystic ovary syndrome (PCOS) and Cushing's syndrome can cause hormonal imbalances that affect insulin sensitivity.

b. Metabolic Syndrome:

A cluster of conditions, including high blood pressure, high blood sugar, excess body fat around the waist, and abnormal cholesterol levels, collectively increase the risk of insulin resistance.

Chronic Inflammation

Chronic low-grade inflammation is often present in individuals with obesity and can contribute to insulin resistance. Adipose tissue, especially visceral fat, secretes inflammatory cytokines that impair insulin signaling pathways.

Cellular Mechanisms

a. Insulin Signaling Pathway Disruption:

Normally, insulin binds to receptors on cell surfaces, triggering a cascade of events that allow glucose to enter cells. In insulin resistance, this signaling pathway is disrupted, possibly due to defects in insulin receptors or post-receptor signaling defects.

b. Lipotoxicity:

Accumulation of fatty acids and their metabolites in non-adipose tissues (such as liver and muscle) can impair insulin signaling and glucose metabolism, contributing to insulin resistance.

Environmental and External Factors

a. Stress:

Chronic stress elevates cortisol levels, a hormone that can increase blood sugar and contribute to insulin resistance.

b. Sleep Patterns:

Poor sleep quality and irregular sleep patterns can affect insulin sensitivity. Sleep deprivation is associated with increased hunger and calorie intake, contributing to weight gain and insulin resistance.

Age and Development

a. Aging:

As individuals age, the risk of insulin resistance increases due to changes in body composition, hormonal shifts, and potential decreases in physical activity.

b. Developmental Factors:

Conditions during pregnancy, such as gestational diabetes, can predispose both the mother and the child to insulin resistance later in life.

CHAPTER III

FUNCTIONS OF INSULIN

RESISTANCE

Insulin resistance is primarily known for its role in disrupting glucose metabolism, but its functions and implications extend beyond just blood sugar regulation. Here's an overview of the key functions and consequences of insulin resistance:

Impaired Glucose Uptake

a. Muscle Cells:
In healthy individuals, insulin facilitates the uptake of glucose into muscle cells for energy production. In insulin resistance, muscle cells fail to respond effectively to insulin, leading to reduced glucose uptake and higher blood sugar levels.

b. Fat Cells:
Insulin promotes the storage of glucose as fat in adipose tissues. When fat cells become insulin resistant, they release more free fatty acids into the bloodstream, which can further impair insulin sensitivity in other tissues.

c. Liver:
Normally, insulin inhibits glucose production in the liver. Insulin resistance in liver cells leads to unchecked glucose production, contributing to elevated blood sugar levels.

Increased Blood Sugar Levels

When cells do not respond properly to insulin, glucose accumulates in the bloodstream, leading to hyperglycemia. The pancreas compensates by producing more insulin (hyperinsulinemia) in an attempt to lower blood sugar levels, but this is often not sustainable long-term.

Metabolic Dysfunction

a. Dyslipidemia:
Insulin resistance often leads to abnormal lipid levels, including increased triglycerides and decreased HDL (good cholesterol). This contributes to a higher risk of cardiovascular diseases.

b. Increased Fat Storage:
Insulin resistance can promote the accumulation of fat, especially in the abdominal region, which further exacerbates insulin resistance and metabolic syndrome.

Inflammatory Responses

Adipose tissue in individuals with insulin resistance often becomes inflamed. This low-grade chronic inflammation is characterized by the release of pro-inflammatory cytokines, which further impair insulin signaling and contribute to metabolic dysfunction.

Impact on Other Hormones

a. Leptin Resistance:
Insulin resistance is often associated with leptin resistance, which affects the regulation of hunger and energy balance. Leptin resistance can lead to increased appetite and overeating, further worsening obesity and insulin resistance.

b. Hormonal Imbalance:
Conditions like polycystic ovary syndrome (PCOS) are linked to insulin resistance and can cause hormonal imbalances that affect reproductive health and increase the risk of other metabolic disorders.

Increased Risk of Type 2 Diabetes

Persistent insulin resistance can lead to beta-cell dysfunction in the pancreas. Over time, the pancreas is unable to produce sufficient insulin to overcome the resistance, resulting in the development of type 2 diabetes.

Cardiovascular Complications

Insulin resistance is a major risk factor for cardiovascular diseases. The combination of high blood sugar, dyslipidemia, and inflammation damages blood vessels, leading to atherosclerosis, hypertension, and increased risk of heart attack and stroke.

BENEFITS OF An INSULIN RESISTANCE DIET

Following an insulin resistance diet offers numerous core benefits, significantly improving health and reducing the risk of developing serious conditions like type 2 diabetes and cardiovascular diseases. Here are the primary benefits:

1. Improved Insulin Sensitivity

An insulin resistance diet focuses on low glycemic index (GI) foods, high in fiber, which helps maintain stable blood sugar levels. Consuming these foods enhances the body's ability to respond to insulin, reducing the demand on the pancreas and improving overall insulin sensitivity.

2. Better Blood Sugar Control

By avoiding refined sugars and processed carbohydrates, this diet prevents spikes in blood sugar levels. Stable blood sugar levels are crucial for managing insulin resistance and preventing the progression to type 2 diabetes. Regular monitoring and balanced meals ensure consistent glucose levels.

3. Weight Management

A diet rich in whole grains, lean proteins, healthy fats, and vegetables supports weight loss and maintenance. Excess weight, particularly around the abdomen, is a significant risk factor for insulin resistance. Shedding even a small percentage of body weight can dramatically improve insulin sensitivity and reduce health risks.

4. Reduced Inflammation

Chronic low-grade inflammation is a hallmark of insulin resistance and is exacerbated by poor dietary choices. An insulin resistance diet, high in antioxidants and anti-inflammatory foods, helps reduce inflammation. Foods like leafy greens, berries, nuts, and fatty fish are particularly beneficial.

5. Lower Risk of Cardiovascular Diseases

Insulin resistance is closely linked to cardiovascular issues such as high blood pressure, high triglycerides, and low HDL cholesterol. By improving lipid profiles and reducing inflammation, an insulin resistance diet lowers the risk of heart disease, stroke, and other cardiovascular conditions.

6. Enhanced Energy Levels

Stable blood sugar levels translate to more consistent energy throughout the day. The diet's emphasis on balanced meals with complex carbohydrates, proteins, and healthy fats ensures sustained energy release, reducing fatigue and improving overall vitality.

7. Better Digestive Health

High-fiber foods, a staple of the insulin resistance diet, promote healthy digestion and regular bowel movements. Improved gut health is linked to better metabolic outcomes and enhanced insulin sensitivity.

8. Hormonal Balance

Proper nutrition can help balance hormones that regulate appetite, metabolism, and stress. Improved insulin sensitivity aids in better hormonal regulation, reducing issues like leptin resistance and the complications of conditions like polycystic ovary syndrome (PCOS).

Following an insulin resistance diet offers multiple benefits, including improved insulin sensitivity, better blood sugar control, weight management, reduced inflammation, and lower cardiovascular risks. It also enhances energy levels, digestive health, and hormonal balance, contributing to overall well-being. By adopting this diet, individuals can effectively manage insulin resistance and prevent associated health complications.

WHAT TO AVOID

An insulin resistance diet focuses on foods that improve insulin sensitivity, stabilize blood sugar levels, and promote overall health. The Ultimate Insulin Resistance Diet for Beginners emphasizes whole, nutrient-dense foods while avoiding those that can cause blood sugar spikes and exacerbate insulin resistance. Here's a detailed guide on what to eat and what to avoid:

Foods to Eat

1. Low Glycemic Index (GI) Foods
❖ **Whole Grains**: Quinoa, brown rice, barley, oats, and whole wheat products. These grains have a low glycemic index, releasing glucose slowly into the bloodstream and helping to maintain stable blood sugar levels.
❖ **Legumes:** Beans, lentils, and chickpeas are excellent sources of complex carbohydrates and fiber, which slow down glucose absorption.

2. High-Fiber Foods
❖ **Vegetables:** Non-starchy vegetables like leafy greens, broccoli, cauliflower, peppers, and tomatoes. These are low in calories and high in vitamins, minerals, and fiber.
❖ **Fruits:** Berries, apples, pears, and citrus fruits. These fruits have a lower glycemic index and provide essential nutrients and antioxidants.

3. Healthy Fats
❖ **Nuts and Seeds:** Almonds, walnuts, chia seeds, and flaxseeds. These provide healthy fats, fiber, and protein, contributing to satiety and stable blood sugar levels.
❖ **Avocados:** Rich in monounsaturated fats, which can help improve insulin sensitivity.
❖ **Oils:** Olive oil, avocado oil, and coconut oil are good choices for cooking and dressing salads.

4. Lean Proteins
❖ **Fish:** Fatty fish like salmon, mackerel, sardines, and trout are rich in omega-3 fatty acids, which have anti-inflammatory properties.
❖ **Poultry:** Skinless chicken and turkey provide lean protein without excessive saturated fat.
❖ **Plant-Based Proteins:** Tofu, tempeh, and legumes are excellent sources of protein for vegetarians and vegans.

5. Whole Foods
❖ **Minimally Processed Foods:** Foods in their natural state, such as whole fruits, vegetables, nuts, and seeds, are preferable over processed options.

Foods to Avoid

1. Refined Sugars and Carbohydrates
❖ **Sugary Snacks:** Candies, cookies, cakes, and pastries cause rapid spikes in blood sugar and insulin levels.
❖ **Sugary Beverages:** Sodas, fruit juices, and energy drinks are high in added sugars and can quickly elevate blood sugar levels.

2. High-Glycemic Index Foods
❖ **White Bread and Pasta:** Made from refined flour, these foods have a high glycemic index and can cause rapid increases in blood sugar.
❖ **White Rice:** Similar to refined grains, white rice is quickly digested and can lead to blood sugar spikes.

3. Trans Fats
❖ **Processed Foods:** Many processed foods contain trans fats, which can worsen insulin resistance and increase inflammation. Avoid foods like margarine, shortening, and commercially baked goods.
❖ **Fried Foods:** Deep-fried foods often contain unhealthy fats and are high in calories, contributing to weight gain and insulin resistance.

4. High-Saturated Fat Foods
❖ **Red Meat:** Limit consumption of red meats such as beef, pork, and lamb. Choose lean cuts if consumed.
❖ **Full-Fat Dairy:** Whole milk, cheese, and butter are high in saturated fats. Opt for low-fat or fat-free versions instead.

Additional Tips for Optimal Health

1. Portion Control: Even healthy foods can lead to weight gain if consumed in excess. Paying attention to portion sizes helps manage calorie intake and supports weight loss or maintenance.

2. Regular Meals: Eating small, regular meals throughout the day can prevent large fluctuations in blood sugar levels and help maintain consistent energy levels.

3. Hydration: Drinking plenty of water is essential for overall health and can help control appetite and blood sugar levels. Avoid sugary drinks and opt for water, herbal teas, or black coffee instead.

4. Physical Activity: Combine a balanced diet with regular physical activity to enhance insulin sensitivity and overall health. Aim for at least 150 minutes of moderate aerobic activity and two days of strength training per week.

The Ultimate Insulin Resistance Diet for Beginners emphasizes eating whole, nutrient-dense foods that improve insulin sensitivity and stabilize blood sugar levels. By focusing on low glycemic index foods, high-fiber foods, healthy fats, and lean proteins, while avoiding refined sugars, high-glycemic index foods, trans fats, and high-saturated fat foods, individuals can effectively manage insulin resistance and achieve optimal health. Coupled with portion control, regular meals, proper hydration, and physical activity, this dietary approach supports long-term health and well-being.

ROLE OF FOOD IN INSULIN RESISTANCE

Food plays a critical role in the development, management, and potential reversal of insulin resistance. The types of foods consumed can significantly impact blood sugar levels, insulin sensitivity, and overall metabolic health. Here's a detailed examination of the role of food in insulin resistance:

Impact on Blood Sugar Levels

a. High Glycemic Index (GI) Foods:
Foods with a high glycemic index, such as white bread, sugary snacks, and beverages, cause rapid spikes in blood sugar levels. These spikes require the pancreas to release large amounts of insulin to manage the sudden influx of glucose. Over time, this can lead to insulin resistance as cells become less responsive to the hormone.

b. Low Glycemic Index (GI) Foods:
Conversely, foods with a low glycemic index, such as whole grains, legumes, and most fruits and vegetables, release glucose more slowly and steadily into the bloodstream. This gradual release helps maintain stable blood sugar levels and reduces the demand on insulin, promoting better insulin sensitivity.

Influence on Insulin Sensitivity

a. Fiber-Rich Foods:

High-fiber foods, including vegetables, fruits, legumes, and whole grains, slow down digestion and the absorption of glucose. This helps prevent blood sugar spikes and enhances insulin sensitivity. Fiber also promotes satiety, aiding in weight management, which is crucial for improving insulin sensitivity.

b. Healthy Fats:

Consuming healthy fats from sources like avocados, nuts, seeds, and olive oil can improve insulin sensitivity. These fats reduce inflammation and help regulate blood sugar levels. Omega-3 fatty acids, found in fatty fish like salmon and mackerel, have anti-inflammatory properties that further support insulin function.

Effects on Inflammation

a. Anti-Inflammatory Foods:

Chronic inflammation is a key contributor to insulin resistance. Foods rich in antioxidants and anti-inflammatory properties, such as berries, leafy greens, nuts, and seeds, can reduce inflammation and support better insulin signaling.

b. Pro-Inflammatory Foods:

On the other hand, foods high in trans fats, refined sugars, and processed ingredients can increase inflammation, exacerbating insulin resistance. Avoiding these foods is essential for reducing inflammation and improving insulin function.

Role in Weight Management

a. Satiety and Nutrient Density:

Foods that are high in fiber, protein, and healthy fats promote feelings of fullness and reduce overall calorie intake, aiding in weight management. Maintaining a healthy weight is one of the most effective ways to improve insulin sensitivity.

b. Caloric Intake:

Overconsumption of calories, particularly from high-sugar and high-fat foods, can lead to weight gain and increased fat storage, especially around the abdomen. Excess visceral fat is closely linked to insulin resistance.

Hormonal Regulation

a. Leptin and Ghrelin:

Insulin resistance is often associated with hormonal imbalances involving leptin (the hormone that signals fullness) and ghrelin (the hunger hormone). A diet high in refined sugars and fats can disrupt these hormones, leading to increased appetite and overeating.

b. Insulin Levels:

Consistently high insulin levels due to frequent consumption of high-GI foods can lead to a state of hyperinsulinemia, where the body produces more insulin to manage blood sugar levels. Over time, this can contribute to insulin resistance.

Food plays a central role in both the development and management of insulin resistance. Consuming a balanced diet rich in low-GI foods, fiber, healthy fats, and anti-inflammatory ingredients can improve insulin sensitivity, stabilize blood sugar levels, reduce inflammation, and support weight management. Conversely, a diet high in refined sugars, processed foods, and unhealthy fats can lead to blood sugar spikes, chronic inflammation, weight gain, and hormonal imbalances, all of which contribute to insulin resistance. Making informed dietary choices is crucial for preventing and managing insulin resistance and promoting overall metabolic health.

NOTE

CHAPTER IV: MEAL PLAN

Week 1

Day 1
Breakfast: Avocado and Egg Breakfast Bowl
Lunch: Mediterranean Chickpea Salad
Dinner: Baked Lemon Garlic Salmon
Snack: Greek Yogurt with Berries and Almonds

Day 2
Breakfast: Greek Yogurt Parfait with Berries and Nuts
Lunch: Quinoa and Vegetable Soup
Dinner: Grilled Lemon Herb Chicken Breast
Snack: Cucumber and Hummus Bites

Day 3
Breakfast: Spinach and Feta Omelet
Lunch: Spinach and Berry Salad with Grilled Chicken
Dinner: Turkey and Vegetable Stir-Fry
Snack: Baked Sweet Potato Fries

Day 4
Breakfast: Chia Seed Pudding with Almond Milk
Lunch: Chicken and Vegetable Stir-Fry Salad
Dinner: Lemon Garlic Butter Cod
Snack: Spicy Roasted Chickpeas

Day 5
Breakfast: Overnight Oats with Flaxseed and Blueberries
Lunch: Lentil and Vegetable Soup
Dinner: Beef and Broccoli Stir-Fry
Snack: Zucchini Noodles with Pesto

Day 6
Breakfast: Veggie and Turkey Sausage Breakfast Skillet
Lunch: Mediterranean Chickpea Salad
Dinner: Pan-Seared Scallops with Garlic Herb Butter
Snack: Greek Yogurt with Berries and Almonds

Day 7
Breakfast: Smoked Salmon and Avocado Toast
Lunch: Quinoa and Vegetable Soup
Dinner: Lemon Herb Roasted Chicken Thighs
Snack: Cucumber and Hummus Bites

Week 2

Day 8
Breakfast: Sweet Potato Hash with Poached Eggs
Lunch: Spinach and Berry Salad with Grilled Chicken
Dinner: Oven-Baked Lemon Herb Tilapia
Snack: Spicy Roasted Chickpeas

Day 9
Breakfast: Coconut Flour Pancakes
Lunch: Chicken and Vegetable Stir-Fry Salad
Dinner: Pork Tenderloin with Balsamic Glaze
Snack: Greek Yogurt with Berries and Almonds

Day 10
Breakfast: Green Smoothie Bowl
Lunch: Mediterranean Chickpea Salad
Dinner: Grilled Shrimp Skewers with Herb Marinade
Snack: Baked Sweet Potato Fries

Day 11
Breakfast: Avocado and Egg Breakfast Bowl
Lunch: Quinoa and Vegetable Soup
Dinner: Lemon Garlic Butter Cod
Snack: Zucchini Noodles with Pesto

Day 12
Breakfast: Greek Yogurt Parfait with Berries and Nuts
Lunch: Lentil and Vegetable Soup
Dinner: Turkey and Vegetable Stir-Fry
Snack: Spicy Roasted Chickpeas

Day 13
Breakfast: Spinach and Feta Omelet
Lunch: Spinach and Berry Salad with Grilled Chicken
Dinner: Pan-Seared Scallops with Garlic Herb Butter
Snack: Greek Yogurt with Berries and Almonds

Day 14
Breakfast: Chia Seed Pudding with Almond Milk
Lunch: Chicken and Vegetable Stir-Fry Salad
Dinner: Beef and Broccoli Stir-Fry
Snack: Cucumber and Hummus Bites

Week 3

Day 15
Breakfast: Overnight Oats with Flaxseed and Blueberries
Lunch: Mediterranean Chickpea Salad
Dinner: Lemon Herb Roasted Chicken Thighs
Snack: Baked Sweet Potato Fries

Day 16
Breakfast: Veggie and Turkey Sausage Breakfast Skillet
Lunch: Quinoa and Vegetable Soup
Dinner: Oven-Baked Lemon Herb Tilapia
Snack: Spicy Roasted Chickpeas

Day 17
Breakfast: Smoked Salmon and Avocado Toast
Lunch: Spinach and Berry Salad with Grilled Chicken
Dinner: Pork Tenderloin with Balsamic Glaze
Snack: Greek Yogurt with Berries and Almonds

Day 18
Breakfast: Sweet Potato Hash with Poached Eggs
Lunch: Chicken and Vegetable Stir-Fry Salad
Dinner: Grilled Shrimp Skewers with Herb Marinade
Snack: Cucumber and Hummus Bites

Day 19
Breakfast: Coconut Flour Pancakes
Lunch: Lentil and Vegetable Soup
Dinner: Lemon Garlic Butter Cod
Snack: Zucchini Noodles with Pesto

Day 20
Breakfast: Green Smoothie Bowl
Lunch: Mediterranean Chickpea Salad
Dinner: Beef and Broccoli Stir-Fry
Snack: Spicy Roasted Chickpeas

Day 21
Breakfast: Avocado and Egg Breakfast Bowl
Lunch: Quinoa and Vegetable Soup
Dinner: Lemon Herb Roasted Chicken Thighs
Snack: Greek Yogurt with Berries and Almonds

Week 4

Day 22
Breakfast: Greek Yogurt Parfait with Berries and Nuts
Lunch: Spinach and Berry Salad with Grilled Chicken
Dinner: Pan-Seared Scallops with Garlic Herb Butter
Snack: Baked Sweet Potato Fries

Day 23
Breakfast: Spinach and Feta Omelet
Lunch: Chicken and Vegetable Stir-Fry Salad
Dinner: Turkey and Vegetable Stir-Fry
Snack: Cucumber and Hummus Bites

Day 24
Breakfast: Chia Seed Pudding with Almond Milk
Lunch: Mediterranean Chickpea Salad
Dinner: Oven-Baked Lemon Herb Tilapia
Snack: Spicy Roasted Chickpeas

Day 25
Breakfast: Overnight Oats with Flaxseed and Blueberries
Lunch: Quinoa and Vegetable Soup
Dinner: Beef and Broccoli Stir-Fry
Snack: Greek Yogurt with Berries and Almonds

Day 26
Breakfast: Veggie and Turkey Sausage Breakfast Skillet
Lunch: Lentil and Vegetable Soup
Dinner: Pork Tenderloin with Balsamic Glaze
Snack: Baked Sweet Potato Fries

Day 27
Breakfast: Smoked Salmon and Avocado Toast
Lunch: Spinach and Berry Salad with Grilled Chicken
Dinner: Lemon Garlic Butter Cod
Snack: Zucchini Noodles with Pesto

Day 28
Breakfast: Sweet Potato Hash with Poached Eggs
Lunch: Chicken and Vegetable Stir-Fry Salad
Dinner: Grilled Shrimp Skewers with Herb Marinade
Snack: Greek Yogurt with Berries and Almonds

LIST OF INGREDIENTS

Vegetables

- Spinach
- Feta Cheese (if considering it a salad addition)
- Sweet Potatoes
- Zucchini
- Bell Peppers
- Cucumber
- Tomatoes
- Carrots
- Broccoli
- Eggplant
- Chickpeas
- Garlic
- Ginger
- Mixed Vegetables (for various stir-fries)
- Scallions
- Basil
- Turmeric

Fish and Seafood

- Salmon
- Shrimp
- Cod
- Scallops
- Tilapia

Dairy and Alternatives

- Greek Yogurt
- Almond Milk
- Feta Cheese (also listed under vegetables for spinach and feta omelet)

Fruits

- Berries (for parfaits, smoothies, salads, and snacks)
- Blueberries
- Strawberries
- Raspberries
- Apples
- Avocado
- Lemon
- Lime

Grains and Legumes

- Quinoa
- Lentils
- Chickpeas (also under vegetables)
- Flaxseed

Poultry and Meat

- Chicken Breast
- Turkey Sausage
- Turkey
- Beef
- Pork Tenderloin

Condiments and Sauces

- Pesto Sauce
- Balsamic Glaze
- Lemon Herb Dressing
- Turmeric Ginger Dressing
- Homemade Tomato Sauce
- Olive Oil
- Salt
- Pepper
- Spices (cinnamon, cumin, turmeric, ginger, etc.)
- Fresh Herb Butter (for seafood dishes)

Nuts and Seeds

- Chia Seeds
- Nuts (for parfaits and snacks)
- Flaxseed

Other Ingredients

- Eggs
- Coconut Flour
- Almond Flour (if using as an alternative to coconut flour)
- Coconut Milk
- Almond Milk
- Hummus
- Pesto (for zucchini noodles)
- Butter (for various cooking methods)
- Lemon Herb Butter (for seafood dishes)

CHAPTER V

BREAKFAST

RECIPES

Avocado and Egg Breakfast Bowl

This avocado and egg breakfast bowl is packed with healthy fats, fiber, and protein, making it an excellent choice for stabilizing blood sugar levels and improving insulin sensitivity.

INGREDIENTS

- ➤ 1 ripe avocado
- ➤ 2 large eggs
- ➤ 1/2 cup cherry tomatoes, halved
- ➤ 1/4 cup red onion, finely chopped
- ➤ 1 tablespoon olive oil
- ➤ 1 tablespoon fresh lemon juice
- ➤ Salt and pepper to taste
- ➤ Fresh cilantro or parsley for garnish

PREPARATION INSTRUCTIONS

1. Slice the avocado in half, remove the pit, and scoop out the flesh into a bowl. Mash it with a fork until smooth.
2. Heat a non-stick pan over medium heat and add the olive oil.
3. Crack the eggs into the pan and cook until the whites are set but the yolks are still runny, about 4-5 minutes.
4. In a small bowl, combine the cherry tomatoes, red onion, and lemon juice. Season with salt and pepper.
5. Divide the mashed avocado between two bowls. Top each with a fried egg.
6. Spoon the tomato mixture around the egg and avocado.
7. Garnish with fresh cilantro or parsley.

NUTRITIONAL VALUE
Calories: 340
Protein: 14g
Carbohydrates: 12g
Fiber: 8g
Fat: 27g

Greek Yogurt Parfait with Berries and Nuts

This Greek yogurt parfait is a simple yet delicious way to start your day. It's rich in protein and fiber, which helps maintain stable blood sugar levels.

INGREDIENTS

- ➤ 1 cup plain Greek yogurt
- ➤ 1/2 cup mixed berries (strawberries, blueberries, raspberries)
- ➤ 1/4 cup granola (low sugar)
- ➤ 2 tablespoons chopped nuts (almonds, walnuts)
- ➤ 1 tablespoon chia seeds
- ➤ 1 tablespoon honey (optional)

PREPARATION INSTRUCTIONS

1. In a glass or bowl, layer half of the Greek yogurt.
2. Add a layer of mixed berries.
3. Sprinkle with half of the granola and chopped nuts.
4. Add the remaining yogurt on top.
5. Finish with the remaining berries, granola, and nuts.
6. Sprinkle chia seeds on top.
7. Drizzle with honey if desired.

NUTRITIONAL VALUE

Calories: 350
Protein: 20g
Carbohydrates: 34g
Fiber: 8g
Fat: 14g

Spinach and Feta Omelet

This spinach and feta omelet is rich in protein and low in carbohydrates, making it a great option for those looking to improve insulin sensitivity.

INGREDIENTS

- ➢ 3 large eggs
- ➢ 1/2 cup fresh spinach, chopped
- ➢ 1/4 cup feta cheese, crumbled
- ➢ 1 tablespoon olive oil
- ➢ Salt and pepper to taste

PREPARATION INSTRUCTIONS

1. In a bowl, whisk the eggs with a pinch of salt and pepper.
2. Heat olive oil in a non-stick skillet over medium heat.
3. Add the chopped spinach and sauté until wilted, about 2 minutes.
4. Pour the beaten eggs over the spinach.
5. Cook until the eggs start to set, then sprinkle the feta cheese over one half of the omelet.
6. Fold the omelet in half and cook for another minute, until the cheese melts.
7. Slide the omelet onto a plate and serve hot.

NUTRITIONAL VALUE

Calories: 280
Protein: 18g
Carbohydrates: 3g
Fiber: 1g
Fat: 22g

Chia Seed Pudding with Almond Milk

Chia seed pudding is an easy, make-ahead breakfast that's high in fiber and omega-3 fatty acids, helping to keep your blood sugar stable throughout the morning.

INGREDIENTS

- 1/4 cup chia seeds
- 1 cup unsweetened almond milk
- 1 tablespoon maple syrup or honey
- 1/2 teaspoon vanilla extract
- Fresh berries for topping

PREPARATION INSTRUCTIONS

1. In a bowl or jar, combine chia seeds, almond milk, maple syrup or honey, and vanilla extract.
2. Stir well to combine.
3. Cover and refrigerate for at least 4 hours or overnight, until the mixture thickens to a pudding-like consistency.
4. Stir the pudding again before serving.
5. Top with fresh berries.

NUTRITIONAL VALUE

Calories: 220
Protein: 6g
Carbohydrates: 20g
Fiber: 12g
Fat: 12g

Overnight Oats with Flaxseed and Blueberries

Overnight oats are a convenient and nutritious breakfast option. This version with flaxseed and blueberries is high in fiber and omega-3 fatty acids, promoting better insulin sensitivity.

INGREDIENTS

- ➤ 1/2 cup rolled oats
- ➤ 1/2 cup unsweetened almond milk
- ➤ 1/4 cup Greek yogurt
- ➤ 1 tablespoon ground flaxseed
- ➤ 1/2 cup blueberries
- ➤ 1 tablespoon honey or maple syrup (optional)
- ➤ 1/2 teaspoon vanilla extract

PREPARATION INSTRUCTIONS

1. In a jar or bowl, combine rolled oats, almond milk, Greek yogurt, ground flaxseed, and vanilla extract.
2. Stir well to mix.
3. Gently fold in the blueberries.
4. Cover and refrigerate overnight.
5. In the morning, stir the oats and add honey or maple syrup if desired.
6. Enjoy cold or warm up in the microwave.

NUTRITIONAL VALUE

Calories: 300
Protein: 10g
Carbohydrates: 45g
Fiber: 8g
Fat: 8g

Veggie and Turkey Sausage Breakfast Skillet

This hearty breakfast skillet is packed with protein and fiber from vegetables and lean turkey sausage, making it a satisfying and balanced meal to start the day.

INGREDIENTS

- ➢ 4 turkey sausage links, sliced
- ➢ 1 red bell pepper, diced
- ➢ 1 green bell pepper, diced
- ➢ 1 small onion, diced
- ➢ 2 cups baby spinach
- ➢ 4 eggs
- ➢ 1 tablespoon olive oil
- ➢ Salt and pepper to taste

PREPARATION INSTRUCTIONS

1. Heat olive oil in a large skillet over medium heat.
2. Add the turkey sausage slices and cook until browned, about 5 minutes.
3. Add the diced bell peppers and onion to the skillet. Cook until vegetables are tender, about 5-7 minutes.
4. Stir in the baby spinach and cook until wilted.
5. Create 4 wells in the vegetable mixture and crack an egg into each well.
6. Cover the skillet and cook until the eggs are cooked to your liking, about 5-7 minutes for runny yolks.
7. Season with salt and pepper.
8. Serve hot, dividing the skillet contents evenly among plates.

NUTRITIONAL VALUE

Calories: 320
Protein: 24g
Carbohydrates: 10g
Fiber: 3g
Fat: 20g

Smoked Salmon and Avocado Toast

This smoked salmon and avocado toast is a delicious combination of healthy fats, protein, and fiber, perfect for a quick and nutritious breakfast.

INGREDIENTS

- ➤ 2 slices whole grain bread, toasted
- ➤ 1 avocado, mashed
- ➤ 4 oz smoked salmon
- ➤ 1 tablespoon capers
- ➤ Fresh dill or parsley for garnish
- ➤ Lemon wedges for serving

PREPARATION INSTRUCTIONS

1. Spread mashed avocado evenly over the toasted bread slices.
2. Top each slice with smoked salmon.
3. Sprinkle capers over the salmon.
4. Garnish with fresh dill or parsley.
5. Serve with lemon wedges for squeezing over the toast.

NUTRITIONAL VALUE

Calories: 380
Protein: 25g
Carbohydrates: 25g
Fiber: 10g
Fat: 20g

Sweet Potato Hash with Poached Eggs

This sweet potato hash is a nutrient-dense breakfast option, combining complex carbohydrates from sweet potatoes with protein-packed poached eggs.

INGREDIENTS

- ➤ 2 medium sweet potatoes, peeled and diced
- ➤ 1 red bell pepper, diced
- ➤ 1 onion, diced
- ➤ 2 cloves garlic, minced
- ➤ 4 eggs
- ➤ 2 tablespoons olive oil
- ➤ Salt and pepper to taste
- ➤ Fresh parsley for garnish

PREPARATION INSTRUCTIONS

1. Heat olive oil in a large skillet over medium heat.
2. Add diced sweet potatoes and cook until slightly softened, about 8-10 minutes.
3. Add bell pepper, onion, and garlic to the skillet. Cook until vegetables are tender and sweet potatoes are cooked through, about 5-7 minutes.
4. Season with salt and pepper.
5. Meanwhile, poach the eggs in a separate pot of simmering water until whites are set but yolks are still runny, about 3-4 minutes.
6. Divide the sweet potato hash among plates.
7. Top each serving with a poached egg.
8. Garnish with fresh parsley.

NUTRITIONAL VALUE

Calories: 350
Protein: 14g
Carbohydrates: 40g
Fiber: 8g
Fat: 16g

Coconut Flour Pancakes

These coconut flour pancakes are gluten-free and low in carbohydrates, making them a suitable option for those managing insulin resistance.

- 1/2 cup coconut flour
- 4 eggs
- 1/2 cup unsweetened almond milk
- 2 tablespoons coconut oil, melted
- 1 tablespoon honey or maple syrup (optional)
- 1/2 teaspoon baking powder
- 1/4 teaspoon salt
- Fresh berries for serving

1. In a bowl, whisk together coconut flour, baking powder, and salt.
2. In a separate bowl, whisk together eggs, almond milk, melted coconut oil, and honey or maple syrup.
3. Gradually add the wet ingredients to the dry ingredients, stirring until smooth.
4. Heat a non-stick skillet or griddle over medium heat and lightly grease with coconut oil.
5. Pour 1/4 cup of batter onto the skillet for each pancake.
6. Cook until bubbles form on the surface, then flip and cook until golden brown on the other side.
7. Serve warm with fresh berries.

NUTRITIONAL VALUE
Calories: 280
Protein: 10g
Carbohydrates: 20g
Fiber: 8g
Fat: 16g

Green Smoothie Bowl

A green smoothie bowl is a refreshing and nutrient-packed breakfast option, rich in antioxidants, fiber, and vitamins to support overall health and insulin sensitivity.

INGREDIENTS

- 1 cup spinach or kale
- 1/2 avocado
- 1/2 cup frozen berries (such as blueberries or raspberries)
- 1/2 cup unsweetened almond milk
- 1 tablespoon chia seeds
- 1 tablespoon almond butter

Optional toppings: sliced banana, shredded coconut, granola

PREPARATION INSTRUCTIONS

1. In a blender, combine spinach or kale, avocado, frozen berries, almond milk, chia seeds, and almond butter.
2. Blend until smooth and creamy, adding more almond milk if needed to reach desired consistency.
3. Pour into a bowl.
4. Top with sliced banana, shredded coconut, and granola if desired.

NUTRITIONAL VALUE
Calories: 300
Protein: 10g
Carbohydrates: 25g
Fiber: 12g
Fat: 18g

NOTE

SOUPS AND SALADS

Quinoa and Vegetable Soup

This quinoa and vegetable soup is hearty, packed with fiber, and low in glycemic index, making it an excellent choice for stabilizing blood sugar levels and promoting satiety.

INGREDIENTS

- 1/2 cup quinoa, rinsed
- 4 cups low-sodium vegetable broth
- 1 carrot, diced
- 1 celery stalk, diced
- 1 onion, diced
- 1 bell pepper, diced
- 2 cloves garlic, minced
- 1 teaspoon dried thyme
- 1 teaspoon dried oregano
- Salt and pepper to taste
- Fresh parsley for garnish

PREPARATION INSTRUCTIONS

1. In a large pot, heat a drizzle of olive oil over medium heat.
2. Add diced onion, carrot, celery, bell pepper, and garlic. Sauté for 5-7 minutes until vegetables are softened.
3. Add quinoa, dried thyme, and dried oregano to the pot. Stir to combine.
4. Pour in vegetable broth and bring to a boil.
5. Reduce heat to low, cover, and simmer for 15-20 minutes until quinoa is cooked and vegetables are tender.
6. Season with salt and pepper to taste.
7. Ladle soup into bowls and garnish with fresh parsley before serving.

NUTRITIONAL VALUE

Calories: 220
Protein: 7g
Carbohydrates: 40g
Fiber: 6g
Fat: 4g

Mediterranean Chickpea Salad

This Mediterranean chickpea salad is refreshing and packed with fiber, protein, and healthy fats, making it a nutritious option for a light lunch or dinner.

INGREDIENTS

- ➤ 1 can (15 oz) chickpeas, drained and rinsed
- ➤ 1 cucumber, diced
- ➤ 1 cup cherry tomatoes, halved
- ➤ 1/4 cup red onion, thinly sliced
- ➤ 1/4 cup Kalamata olives, pitted and sliced
- ➤ 1/4 cup crumbled feta cheese
- ➤ 2 tablespoons extra virgin olive oil
- ➤ 1 tablespoon red wine vinegar
- ➤ 1 teaspoon dried oregano
- ➤ Salt and pepper to taste
- ➤ Fresh parsley for garnish

PREPARATION INSTRUCTIONS

1. In a large bowl, combine chickpeas, cucumber, cherry tomatoes, red onion, Kalamata olives, and feta cheese.
2. In a small bowl, whisk together olive oil, red wine vinegar, dried oregano, salt, and pepper.
3. Pour the dressing over the salad ingredients and toss gently to coat.
4. Garnish with fresh parsley before serving.

NUTRITIONAL VALUE
Calories: 320
Protein: 12g
Carbohydrates: 30g
Fiber: 8g
Fat: 18g

Chicken and Vegetable Stir-Fry Salad

This chicken and vegetable stir-fry salad is packed with lean protein and fiber-rich vegetables, providing a satisfying meal that supports stable blood sugar levels.

INGREDIENTS

- 2 boneless, skinless chicken breasts, sliced
- 1 red bell pepper, thinly sliced
- 1 yellow bell pepper, thinly sliced
- 1 cup snow peas
- 1 carrot, julienned
- 2 cups shredded cabbage (green or purple)
- 2 tablespoons low-sodium soy sauce
- 1 tablespoon sesame oil
- 1 tablespoon rice vinegar
- 1 teaspoon honey (optional)
- 2 tablespoons sesame seeds
- Fresh cilantro or green onions for garnish

PREPARATION INSTRUCTIONS

1. Heat sesame oil in a large skillet or wok over medium-high heat.
2. Add sliced chicken breasts and cook until browned and cooked through, about 5-7 minutes.
3. Add bell peppers, snow peas, and julienned carrot to the skillet. Stir-fry for another 3-4 minutes until vegetables are tender-crisp.
4. In a small bowl, whisk together soy sauce, rice vinegar, and honey (if using).
5. Pour the sauce over the chicken and vegetables in the skillet. Stir to coat evenly.
6. Remove from heat and let cool slightly.
7. In a large bowl, combine shredded cabbage with the chicken and vegetable mixture.
8. Sprinkle sesame seeds over the salad and toss gently to combine.
9. Garnish with fresh cilantro or green onions before serving.

NUTRITIONAL VALUE
Calories: 380
Protein: 30g
Carbohydrates: 20g
Fiber: 6g
Fat: 20g

Spinach and Berry Salad with Grilled Chicken

This spinach and berry salad with grilled chicken is loaded with antioxidants, fiber, and lean protein, offering a delicious and nutritious option for a light meal.

INGREDIENTS

- 2 boneless, skinless chicken breasts
- 4 cups fresh baby spinach
- 1 cup mixed berries (strawberries, blueberries, raspberries)
- 1/4 cup sliced almonds
- 1/4 cup crumbled goat cheese
- 2 tablespoons balsamic vinegar
- 1 tablespoon extra-virgin olive oil
- 1 teaspoon honey (optional)
- Salt and pepper to taste

PREPARATION INSTRUCTIONS

1. Preheat grill or grill pan over medium-high heat.
2. Season chicken breasts with salt and pepper.
3. Grill chicken breasts for 6-7 minutes per side until cooked through and juices run clear.
4. Remove chicken from grill and let rest for 5 minutes before slicing.
5. In a large bowl, combine baby spinach, mixed berries, sliced almonds, and crumbled goat cheese.
6. In a small bowl, whisk together balsamic vinegar, olive oil, and honey (if using).
7. Drizzle the dressing over the salad and toss gently to coat.
8. Divide the salad onto plates and top with sliced grilled chicken.

NUTRITIONAL VALUE

Calories: 350
Protein: 30g
Carbohydrates: 20g
Fiber: 6g
Fat: 18g

Lentil and Vegetable Soup

This lentil and vegetable soup is rich in fiber, protein, and essential nutrients, providing a satisfying and nutritious meal option that supports stable blood sugar levels.

INGREDIENTS

- 1 cup dried green or brown lentils, rinsed
- 4 cups low-sodium vegetable broth
- 1 onion, diced
- 2 carrots, diced
- 2 celery stalks, diced
- 2 cloves garlic, minced
- 1 teaspoon ground cumin
- 1/2 teaspoon ground turmeric
- 1 bay leaf
- Salt and pepper to taste
- Fresh parsley or cilantro for garnish

PREPARATION INSTRUCTIONS

1. In a large pot, heat a drizzle of olive oil over medium heat.
2. Add diced onion, carrots, celery, and garlic. Sauté for 5-7 minutes until vegetables are softened.
3. Add lentils, ground cumin, ground turmeric, and bay leaf to the pot. Stir to combine.
4. Pour in vegetable broth and bring to a boil.
5. Reduce heat to low, cover, and simmer for 20-25 minutes until lentils are tender.
6. Season with salt and pepper to taste.
7. Remove bay leaf before serving.
8. Ladle soup into bowls and garnish with fresh parsley or cilantro.

NUTRITIONAL VALUE
Calories: 300
Protein: 18g
Carbohydrates: 50g
Fiber: 15g
Fat: 2g

SNACKS AND SIDES

Cucumber and Hummus Bites

These cucumber and hummus bites are a refreshing and satisfying snack, providing fiber, healthy fats, and protein to support stable blood sugar levels.

INGREDIENTS

- ➤ 1 large cucumber, cut into rounds
- ➤ 1/2 cup hummus (store-bought or homemade)
- ➤ Cherry tomatoes, sliced (for garnish)
- ➤ Fresh parsley or dill (for garnish)

PREPARATION INSTRUCTIONS

1. Slice the cucumber into rounds, about 1/4 inch thick.
2. Spoon a small dollop of hummus onto each cucumber round.
3. Garnish each bite with a slice of cherry tomato and a sprig of fresh parsley or dill.
4. Arrange on a serving platter and serve immediately.

NUTRITIONAL VALUE

Calories: 80
Protein: 4g
Carbohydrates: 8g
Fiber: 3g
Fat: 4g

Baked Sweet Potato Fries

These baked sweet potato fries are a healthier alternative to traditional fries, providing complex carbohydrates, fiber, and essential vitamins and minerals.

INGREDIENTS

- ➢ 2 medium sweet potatoes, peeled and cut into fries
- ➢ 2 tablespoons olive oil
- ➢ 1 teaspoon paprika
- ➢ 1/2 teaspoon garlic powder
- ➢ Salt and pepper to taste

PREPARATION INSTRUCTIONS

1. Preheat oven to 425°F (220°C). Line a baking sheet with parchment paper.
2. In a large bowl, toss sweet potato fries with olive oil, paprika, garlic powder, salt, and pepper until evenly coated.
3. Spread the fries in a single layer on the prepared baking sheet.
4. Bake for 20-25 minutes, flipping halfway through, until fries are golden brown and crispy.
5. Remove from oven and let cool slightly before serving.

NUTRITIONAL VALUE
Calories: 180
Protein: 2g
Carbohydrates: 28g
Fiber: 4g
Fat: 7g

Greek Yogurt with Berries and Almonds

Greek yogurt with berries and almonds is a nutritious snack rich in protein, fiber, and healthy fats, supporting stable blood sugar levels and promoting satiety.

INGREDIENTS

- 1 cup plain Greek yogurt
- 1/2 cup mixed berries (such as strawberries, blueberries, raspberries)
- 1/4 cup almonds, chopped
- 1 tablespoon honey (optional)

PREPARATION INSTRUCTIONS

1. In a bowl, spoon Greek yogurt.
2. Top with mixed berries and chopped almonds.
3. Drizzle with honey if desired.
4. Serve immediately.

NUTRITIONAL VALUE

Calories: 280
Protein: 20g
Carbohydrates: 20g
Fiber: 5g
Fat: 15g

Zucchini Noodles with Pesto

Zucchini noodles with pesto are a low-carb and nutrient-dense side dish, providing fiber, vitamins, minerals, and healthy fats.

INGREDIENTS

- ➢ 2 large zucchinis, spiralized into noodles
- ➢ 1/4 cup homemade or store-bought pesto
- ➢ Cherry tomatoes, halved (for garnish)
- ➢ Grated Parmesan cheese (optional, for garnish)

PREPARATION INSTRUCTIONS

1. Spiralize zucchinis into noodles using a spiralizer or julienne peeler.
2. Heat a large skillet over medium heat.
3. Add zucchini noodles and cook for 2-3 minutes until just tender.
4. Remove from heat and toss with pesto until noodles are evenly coated.
5. Garnish with cherry tomatoes and grated Parmesan cheese if desired.
6. Serve warm or at room temperature.

NUTRITIONAL VALUE
Calories: 180
Protein: 5g
Carbohydrates: 10g
Fiber: 3g
Fat: 14g

Spicy Roasted Chickpeas

Spicy roasted chickpeas are a crunchy and protein-rich snack, providing fiber and essential nutrients while satisfying cravings for something savory.

INGREDIENTS

- ➤ 1 can (15 oz) chickpeas, drained, rinsed, and patted dry
- ➤ 1 tablespoon olive oil
- ➤ 1 teaspoon paprika
- ➤ 1/2 teaspoon cumin
- ➤ 1/2 teaspoon garlic powder
- ➤ Salt and pepper to taste

PREPARATION INSTRUCTIONS

1. Preheat oven to 400°F (200°C). Line a baking sheet with parchment paper.
2. In a bowl, toss chickpeas with olive oil, paprika, cumin, garlic powder, salt, and pepper until evenly coated.
3. Spread chickpeas in a single layer on the prepared baking sheet.
4. Bake for 25-30 minutes, shaking the pan halfway through, until chickpeas are crispy and golden brown.
5. Remove from oven and let cool before serving.

NUTRITIONAL VALUE
Calories: 160
Protein: 6g
Carbohydrates: 20g
Fiber: 5g
Fat: 6g

VEGETARIAN AND VEGAN

Quinoa Stuffed Bell Peppers

Quinoa stuffed bell peppers are a nutrient-dense and satisfying vegetarian meal, rich in fiber, protein, and essential vitamins and minerals.

INGREDIENTS

- ➤ 4 large bell peppers (any color)
- ➤ 1 cup quinoa, rinsed
- ➤ 2 cups vegetable broth
- ➤ 1 can (15 oz) black beans, drained and rinsed
- ➤ 1 cup corn kernels (fresh or frozen)
- ➤ 1 cup diced tomatoes (canned or fresh)
- ➤ 1 teaspoon cumin
- ➤ 1/2 teaspoon chili powder
- ➤ Salt and pepper to taste
- ➤ Fresh cilantro for garnish

PREPARATION INSTRUCTIONS

1. Preheat oven to 375°F (190°C). Grease a baking dish with olive oil.
2. Cut the tops off the bell peppers and remove seeds and membranes.
3. In a medium saucepan, bring vegetable broth to a boil. Add quinoa, reduce heat to low, cover, and simmer for 15 minutes or until quinoa is cooked and liquid is absorbed.
4. In a large bowl, combine cooked quinoa, black beans, corn, diced tomatoes, cumin, chili powder, salt, and pepper.
5. Spoon the quinoa mixture evenly into each bell pepper.
6. Place stuffed peppers in the prepared baking dish. Cover with foil and bake for 30-35 minutes until peppers are tender.
7. Remove foil and bake for an additional 5 minutes to lightly brown the tops.
8. Garnish with fresh cilantro before serving.

NUTRITIONAL VALUE

Calories: 320
Protein: 12g
Carbohydrates: 60g
Fiber: 12g
Fat: 5g

Lentil Spinach Curry

Lentil spinach curry is a flavorful and protein-packed vegetarian dish, rich in fiber and essential nutrients, perfect for maintaining stable blood sugar levels.

INGREDIENTS

- 1 cup dried lentils (green or brown), rinsed
- 4 cups vegetable broth
- 1 onion, diced
- 2 cloves garlic, minced
- 1 tablespoon grated fresh ginger
- 1 tablespoon curry powder
- 1 teaspoon ground turmeric
- 1 can (14 oz) diced tomatoes
- 4 cups fresh spinach leaves
- Salt and pepper to taste
- Fresh cilantro for garnish

PREPARATION INSTRUCTIONS

1. In a large pot, heat a drizzle of olive oil over medium heat.
2. Add diced onion and cook until translucent, about 5 minutes.
3. Add minced garlic, grated ginger, curry powder, and ground turmeric. Cook for 1 minute until fragrant.
4. Stir in dried lentils, vegetable broth, and diced tomatoes with their juices. Bring to a boil.
5. Reduce heat to low, cover, and simmer for 20-25 minutes until lentils are tender.
6. Stir in fresh spinach leaves and cook for 2-3 minutes until wilted.
7. Season with salt and pepper to taste.
8. Garnish with fresh cilantro before serving.

NUTRITIONAL VALUE
Calories: 280
Protein: 18g
Carbohydrates: 50g
Fiber: 15g
Fat: 2g

Eggplant and Chickpea Curry

Eggplant and chickpea curry is a hearty and flavorful vegetarian dish, rich in fiber, protein, and antioxidants, supporting stable blood sugar levels and overall health.

INGREDIENTS

- 1 large eggplant, diced
- 1 can (15 oz) chickpeas, drained and rinsed
- 1 onion, diced
- 2 cloves garlic, minced
- 1 tablespoon grated fresh ginger
- 1 tablespoon curry powder
- 1 teaspoon ground cumin
- 1/2 teaspoon ground coriander
- 1 can (14 oz) diced tomatoes
- 1 cup coconut milk (full-fat or light)
- Salt and pepper to taste
- Fresh cilantro for garnish

PREPARATION INSTRUCTIONS

1. Heat a drizzle of olive oil in a large skillet or pot over medium heat.
2. Add diced onion and cook until translucent, about 5 minutes.
3. Add minced garlic, grated ginger, curry powder, ground cumin, and ground coriander. Cook for 1 minute until fragrant.
4. Add diced eggplant and cook for 5-7 minutes until slightly softened.
5. Stir in chickpeas, diced tomatoes with their juices, and coconut milk. Bring to a simmer.
6. Reduce heat to low, cover, and cook for 20-25 minutes until eggplant is tender.
7. Season with salt and pepper to taste.
8. Garnish with fresh cilantro before serving.

NUTRITIONAL VALUE
Calories: 350
Protein: 14g
Carbohydrates: 45g
Fiber: 12g
Fat: 15g

Caprese Salad with Avocado

Caprese salad with avocado is a refreshing and nutrient-rich vegetarian dish, providing healthy fats, vitamins, minerals, and antioxidants to support overall health and stable blood sugar levels.

INGREDIENTS

- ➤ 2 large tomatoes, sliced
- ➤ 1 avocado, sliced
- ➤ 8 oz fresh mozzarella cheese, sliced
- ➤ Fresh basil leaves
- ➤ 2 tablespoons extra virgin olive oil
- ➤ 1 tablespoon balsamic vinegar
- ➤ Salt and pepper to taste

PREPARATION INSTRUCTIONS

1. Arrange sliced tomatoes, avocado, and mozzarella cheese on a serving platter, alternating layers.
2. Tuck fresh basil leaves between the layers.
3. Drizzle with extra virgin olive oil and balsamic vinegar.
4. Season with salt and pepper to taste.
5. Serve immediately as a side dish or light lunch.

NUTRITIONAL VALUE
Calories: 320
Protein: 18g
Carbohydrates: 10g
Fiber: 5g
Fat: 25g

Stir-Fried Tofu with Vegetables

Stir-fried tofu with vegetables is a quick and nutritious vegetarian dish, rich in protein, fiber, and essential nutrients, ideal for maintaining stable blood sugar levels.

INGREDIENTS

- ➤ 1 block (14 oz) firm tofu, drained and cut into cubes
- ➤ 1 bell pepper, thinly sliced
- ➤ 1 zucchini, thinly sliced
- ➤ 1 carrot, julienned
- ➤ 1 cup snow peas
- ➤ 2 tablespoons low-sodium soy sauce
- ➤ 1 tablespoon sesame oil
- ➤ 1 tablespoon rice vinegar
- ➤ 1 teaspoon grated fresh ginger
- ➤ 2 cloves garlic, minced
- ➤ Fresh cilantro or green onions for garnish

PREPARATION INSTRUCTIONS

1. Heat sesame oil in a large skillet or wok over medium-high heat.
2. Add tofu cubes and cook until golden brown on all sides, about 5-7 minutes. Remove tofu from skillet and set aside.
3. In the same skillet, add bell pepper, zucchini, carrot, and snow peas. Stir-fry for 3-4 minutes until vegetables are tender-crisp.
4. Add minced garlic and grated ginger. Cook for 1 minute until fragrant.
5. Return tofu to the skillet.
6. In a small bowl, whisk together soy sauce and rice vinegar. Pour over the tofu and vegetables.
7. Stir-fry for another 2-3 minutes until everything is heated through and evenly coated.
8. Garnish with fresh cilantro or green onions before serving.

NUTRITIONAL VALUE

Calories: 280
Protein: 20g
Carbohydrates: 20g
Fiber: 6g
Fat: 15g

FISH AND SEAFOOD

Baked Lemon Garlic Salmon

Baked lemon garlic salmon is flavorful and nutritious dish rich in omega-3 fatty acids, protein, and essential vitamins and minerals, making it ideal for supporting stable blood sugar levels.

INGREDIENTS

- ➢ 4 salmon fillets (about 6 oz each)
- ➢ 2 tablespoons olive oil
- ➢ 4 cloves garlic, minced
- ➢ Zest and juice of 1 lemon
- ➢ 1 teaspoon dried thyme
- ➢ Salt and pepper to taste
- ➢ Fresh parsley for garnish

PREPARATION INSTRUCTIONS

1. Preheat oven to 400°F (200°C). Line a baking sheet with parchment paper.
2. Place salmon fillets on the prepared baking sheet.
3. In a small bowl, whisk together olive oil, minced garlic, lemon zest, lemon juice, dried thyme, salt, and pepper.
4. Spoon the lemon garlic mixture evenly over the salmon fillets, spreading to coat.
5. Bake for 12-15 minutes, or until salmon is cooked through and flakes easily with a fork.
6. Remove from oven and garnish with fresh parsley before serving.

NUTRITIONAL VALUE
Calories: 350
Protein: 34g
Carbohydrates: 2g
Fiber: 0g
Fat: 22g

Grilled Shrimp Skewers with Herb Marinade

Grilled shrimp skewers with herb marinade are a delicious and low-carb option, packed with protein, antioxidants, and healthy fats, perfect for maintaining stable blood sugar levels.

INGREDIENTS

- ➤ 1 lb large shrimp, peeled and deveined
- ➤ 2 tablespoons olive oil
- ➤ 2 cloves garlic, minced
- ➤ 1 tablespoon chopped fresh parsley
- ➤ 1 tablespoon chopped fresh basil
- ➤ 1 tablespoon chopped fresh thyme
- ➤ Zest and juice of 1 lemon
- ➤ Salt and pepper to taste

PREPARATION INSTRUCTIONS

1. In a bowl, combine olive oil, minced garlic, chopped parsley, basil, thyme, lemon zest, lemon juice, salt, and pepper.
2. Add shrimp to the marinade, tossing to coat evenly. Cover and refrigerate for at least 30 minutes.
3. Preheat grill or grill pan over medium-high heat.
4. Thread shrimp onto skewers, discarding any leftover marinade.
5. Grill shrimp skewers for 2-3 minutes per side, or until shrimp are pink and opaque.
6. Remove from grill and serve immediately.

NUTRITIONAL VALUE
Calories: 200
Protein: 24g
Carbohydrates: 2g
Fiber: 0g
Fat: 11g

Lemon Garlic Butter Cod

Lemon garlic butter cod is a light and flavorful dish, rich in lean protein, omega-3 fatty acids, and essential nutrients, supporting stable blood sugar levels and overall health.

INGREDIENTS

- ➢ 4 cod fillets (about 6 oz each)
- ➢ 4 tablespoons unsalted butter, melted
- ➢ 4 cloves garlic, minced
- ➢ Zest and juice of 1 lemon
- ➢ 1 teaspoon dried parsley
- ➢ Salt and pepper to taste

PREPARATION INSTRUCTIONS

1. Preheat oven to 400°F (200°C). Line a baking sheet with parchment paper.
2. Place cod fillets on the prepared baking sheet.
3. In a small bowl, whisk together melted butter, minced garlic, lemon zest, lemon juice, dried parsley, salt, and pepper.
4. Spoon the lemon garlic butter mixture evenly over the cod fillets, spreading to coat.
5. Bake for 12-15 minutes, or until cod is opaque and flakes easily with a fork.
6. Remove from oven and serve immediately.

NUTRITIONAL VALUE

Calories: 280
Protein: 30g
Carbohydrates: 2g
Fiber: 0g
Fat: 17g

Pan-Seared Scallops with Garlic Herb Butter

Pan-seared scallops with garlic herb butter are a decadent yet healthy seafood dish, rich in protein, omega-3 fatty acids, and essential nutrients, perfect for supporting stable blood sugar levels.

INGREDIENTS

- ➤ 1 lb sea scallops
- ➤ 2 tablespoons unsalted butter
- ➤ 2 cloves garlic, minced
- ➤ 1 tablespoon chopped fresh parsley
- ➤ 1 tablespoon chopped fresh chives
- ➤ Salt and pepper to taste
- ➤ Lemon wedges for serving

PREPARATION INSTRUCTIONS

1. Pat scallops dry with paper towels and season both sides with salt and pepper.
2. In a large skillet, melt butter over medium-high heat.
3. Add minced garlic and cook for 1 minute until fragrant.
4. Add scallops to the skillet in a single layer, making sure not to overcrowd.
5. Sear scallops for 2-3 minutes per side, or until golden brown and opaque.
6. Remove scallops from skillet and transfer to a plate.
7. Stir chopped parsley and chives into the garlic butter remaining in the skillet.
8. Pour the garlic herb butter over the scallops.
9. Serve immediately with lemon wedges on the side.

NUTRITIONAL VALUE

Calories: 250
Protein: 25g
Carbohydrates: 4g
Fiber: 0g
Fat: 14g

Oven-Baked Lemon Herb Tilapia

Oven-baked lemon herb tilapia is a light and flavorful dish, rich in lean protein, omega-3 fatty acids, and essential nutrients, ideal for maintaining stable blood sugar levels.

INGREDIENTS

- ➤ 4 tilapia fillets (about 6 oz each)
- ➤ 2 tablespoons olive oil
- ➤ Zest and juice of 1 lemon
- ➤ 1 teaspoon dried thyme
- ➤ 1 teaspoon dried parsley
- ➤ 1/2 teaspoon garlic powder
- ➤ Salt and pepper to taste

PREPARATION INSTRUCTIONS

1. Preheat oven to 400°F (200°C). Line a baking sheet with parchment paper.
2. Place tilapia fillets on the prepared baking sheet.
3. In a small bowl, whisk together olive oil, lemon zest, lemon juice, dried thyme, dried parsley, garlic powder, salt, and pepper.
4. Spoon the lemon herb mixture evenly over the tilapia fillets, spreading to coat.
5. Bake for 12-15 minutes, or until tilapia is opaque and flakes easily with a fork.
6. Remove from oven and serve immediately.

NUTRITIONAL VALUE
Calories: 220
Protein: 30g
Carbohydrates: 2g
Fiber: 0g
Fat: 10g

POULTRY AND MEAT

Grilled Lemon Herb Chicken Breast

Grilled lemon herb chicken breast is a simple yet flavorful dish, rich in lean protein and essential nutrients, perfect for supporting stable blood sugar levels.

INGREDIENTS

- ➢ 4 boneless, skinless chicken breasts
- ➢ Zest and juice of 1 lemon
- ➢ 2 tablespoons olive oil
- ➢ 2 cloves garlic, minced
- ➢ 1 teaspoon dried thyme
- ➢ 1 teaspoon dried rosemary
- ➢ Salt and pepper to taste
- ➢ Fresh parsley for garnish

PREPARATION INSTRUCTIONS

1. In a bowl, whisk together lemon zest, lemon juice, olive oil, minced garlic, dried thyme, dried rosemary, salt, and pepper.
2. Place chicken breasts in a shallow dish or resealable plastic bag. Pour the marinade over the chicken, turning to coat evenly. Cover or seal and refrigerate for at least 30 minutes, or up to 4 hours.
3. Preheat grill to medium-high heat.
4. Remove chicken from marinade and discard the marinade.
5. Grill chicken breasts for 6-7 minutes per side, or until internal temperature reaches 165°F (74°C) and juices run clear.
6. Remove from grill and let rest for 5 minutes before serving.
7. Garnish with fresh parsley before serving.

NUTRITIONAL VALUE
Calories: 250
Protein: 30g
Carbohydrates: 2g
Fiber: 0g
Fat: 12g

Turkey and Vegetable Stir-Fry

Turkey and vegetable stir-fry is a nutritious and low-carb dish, packed with lean protein, fiber-rich vegetables, and essential nutrients, ideal for managing insulin resistance.

INGREDIENTS

- 1 lb turkey breast, thinly sliced
- 1 tablespoon olive oil
- 1 onion, thinly sliced
- 1 bell pepper, thinly sliced
- 1 zucchini, thinly sliced
- 1 cup snow peas
- 2 cloves garlic, minced
- 1 tablespoon low-sodium soy sauce
- 1 teaspoon sesame oil
- Salt and pepper to taste
- Fresh cilantro or green onions for garnish

PREPARATION INSTRUCTIONS

1. Heat olive oil in a large skillet or wok over medium-high heat.
2. Add thinly sliced turkey breast and cook for 5-6 minutes until browned and cooked through. Remove from skillet and set aside.
3. In the same skillet, add onion, bell pepper, zucchini, and snow peas. Stir-fry for 3-4 minutes until vegetables are tender-crisp.
4. Add minced garlic and cook for 1 minute until fragrant.
5. Return cooked turkey to the skillet.
6. Drizzle low-sodium soy sauce and sesame oil over the turkey and vegetables. Toss to combine.
7. Season with salt and pepper to taste.
8. Garnish with fresh cilantro or green onions before serving.

NUTRITIONAL VALUE
Calories: 280
Protein: 30g
Carbohydrates: 10g
Fiber: 3g
Fat: 12g

Beef and Broccoli Stir-Fry

Beef and broccoli stir-fry is a classic dish made healthier, featuring lean beef, fiber-rich broccoli, and a savory sauce, perfect for those managing insulin resistance.

INGREDIENTS

- 1 lb flank steak, thinly sliced
- 2 tablespoons low-sodium soy sauce
- 1 tablespoon cornstarch
- 1 tablespoon olive oil
- 2 cloves garlic, minced
- 1 tablespoon grated fresh ginger
- 4 cups broccoli florets
- 1/2 cup beef broth (low-sodium)
- 1 tablespoon oyster sauce
- 1 teaspoon sesame oil
- Salt and pepper to taste

PREPARATION INSTRUCTIONS

1. In a bowl, combine thinly sliced flank steak with low-sodium soy sauce and cornstarch. Toss to coat evenly and set aside.
2. Heat olive oil in a large skillet or wok over medium-high heat.
3. Add minced garlic and grated fresh ginger. Cook for 1 minute until fragrant.
4. Add marinated flank steak to the skillet. Stir-fry for 3-4 minutes until beef is browned and cooked through. Remove from skillet and set aside.
5. In the same skillet, add broccoli florets and beef broth. Cover and cook for 3-4 minutes until broccoli is tender-crisp.
6. Return cooked beef to the skillet.
7. Stir in oyster sauce and sesame oil. Toss to combine and heat through.
8. Season with salt and pepper to taste.
9. Serve hot, optionally garnished with sesame seeds.

NUTRITIONAL VALUE

Calories: 320
Protein: 35g
Carbohydrates: 10g
Fiber: 3g
Fat: 15g

Lemon Herb Roasted Chicken Thighs

Lemon herb roasted chicken thighs are a flavorful and satisfying dish, rich in protein and essential nutrients, perfect for supporting stable blood sugar levels.

INGREDIENTS

- 4 chicken thighs, bone-in and skin-on
- Zest and juice of 1 lemon
- 2 tablespoons olive oil
- 2 cloves garlic, minced
- 1 teaspoon dried thyme
- 1 teaspoon dried rosemary
- Salt and pepper to taste
- Fresh parsley for garnish

PREPARATION INSTRUCTIONS

1. Preheat oven to 400°F (200°C). Line a baking sheet with parchment paper.
2. In a bowl, whisk together lemon zest, lemon juice, olive oil, minced garlic, dried thyme, dried rosemary, salt, and pepper.
3. Place chicken thighs on the prepared baking sheet.
4. Spoon the lemon herb mixture evenly over the chicken thighs, spreading to coat.
5. Roast chicken thighs for 30-35 minutes, or until golden brown and cooked through (internal temperature of 165°F or 74°C).
6. Remove from oven and let rest for 5 minutes before serving.
7. Garnish with fresh parsley before serving.

NUTRITIONAL VALUE

Calories: 300
Protein: 25g
Carbohydrates: 0g
Fiber: 0g
Fat: 22g

Pork Tenderloin with Balsamic Glaze

Pork tenderloin with balsamic glaze is a tender and flavorful dish, rich in lean protein and essential nutrients, perfect for those managing insulin resistance.

INGREDIENTS

- ➤ 1 lb pork tenderloin
- ➤ Salt and pepper to taste
- ➤ 1 tablespoon olive oil
- ➤ 1/4 cup balsamic vinegar
- ➤ 2 tablespoons honey (optional)
- ➤ 2 cloves garlic, minced
- ➤ Fresh rosemary or thyme for garnish

PREPARATION INSTRUCTIONS

1. Preheat oven to 400°F (200°C).
2. Season pork tenderloin with salt and pepper.
3. In an oven-safe skillet, heat olive oil over medium-high heat.
4. Sear pork tenderloin on all sides until browned, about 2-3 minutes per side.
5. Transfer skillet to the preheated oven and roast for 15-20 minutes, or until internal temperature reaches 145°F (63°C).
6. Remove pork tenderloin from skillet and let rest on a cutting board, tented with foil, for 5-10 minutes.
7. While pork rests, prepare the balsamic glaze: In the same skillet over medium heat, add balsamic vinegar, honey (if using), and minced garlic. Cook for 2-3 minutes, stirring constantly, until sauce thickens slightly.
8. Slice pork tenderloin and drizzle with balsamic glaze.
9. Garnish with fresh rosemary or thyme before serving.

NUTRITIONAL VALUE

Calories: 250
Protein: 30g
Carbohydrates: 6g
Fiber: 0g
Fat: 10g

DRINK AND DESSERT

Chia Seed Pudding

Chia seed pudding is a nutritious and satisfying dessert or snack, rich in fiber, omega-3 fatty acids, and antioxidants, perfect for managing insulin resistance.

INGREDIENTS

- ➤ 1/4 cup chia seeds
- ➤ 1 cup unsweetened almond milk (or any milk of choice)
- ➤ 1 tablespoon pure maple syrup (optional)
- ➤ 1/2 teaspoon vanilla extract
- ➤ Fresh berries for topping

PREPARATION INSTRUCTIONS

1. In a bowl, combine chia seeds, almond milk, maple syrup (if using), and vanilla extract. Stir well.
2. Cover and refrigerate for at least 2 hours, or overnight, until mixture thickens and chia seeds have absorbed the liquid.
3. Stir the pudding mixture again before serving.
4. Divide into serving bowls or jars, and top with fresh berries.
5. Serve chilled.

NUTRITIONAL VALUE
Calories: 180
Protein: 5g
Carbohydrates: 20g
Fiber: 10g
Fat: 8g

Avocado Chocolate Mousse

Avocado chocolate mousse is a creamy and indulgent dessert, rich in healthy fats, fiber, and antioxidants, suitable for those managing insulin resistance.

INGREDIENTS

- 2 ripe avocados
- 1/4 cup unsweetened cocoa powder
- 1/4 cup pure maple syrup or honey
- 1 teaspoon vanilla extract
- Pinch of salt
- Fresh berries or nuts for garnish

PREPARATION INSTRUCTIONS

1. Scoop the flesh of the avocados into a food processor or blender.
2. Add cocoa powder, maple syrup (or honey), vanilla extract, and a pinch of salt.
3. Blend until smooth and creamy, scraping down the sides as needed.
4. Taste and adjust sweetness if desired, adding more maple syrup or honey.
5. Spoon the avocado chocolate mousse into serving bowls or glasses.
6. Chill in the refrigerator for at least 30 minutes before serving.
7. Garnish with fresh berries or nuts before serving.

NUTRITIONAL VALUE

Calories: 220
Protein: 4g
Carbohydrates: 22g
Fiber: 8g
Fat: 15g

Berry Smoothie

A berry smoothie is a refreshing and nutrient-packed drink, rich in antioxidants, vitamins, and fiber, perfect for a quick and healthy option in an insulin resistance diet.

INGREDIENTS

- ➤ 1 cup mixed berries (strawberries, blueberries, raspberries)
- ➤ 1/2 cup unsweetened Greek yogurt
- ➤ 1/2 cup unsweetened almond milk (or any milk of choice)
- ➤ 1 tablespoon chia seeds
- ➤ 1 teaspoon honey or pure maple syrup (optional)
- ➤ Ice cubes (optional)

PREPARATION INSTRUCTIONS

1. In a blender, combine mixed berries, Greek yogurt, almond milk, chia seeds, and honey or maple syrup (if using).
2. Blend until smooth and creamy.
3. If desired, add ice cubes and blend again until smooth.
4. Pour into glasses and serve immediately.

NUTRITIONAL VALUE
Calories: 180
Protein: 10g
Carbohydrates: 25g
Fiber: 8g
Fat: 5g

Cinnamon Baked Apples

Cinnamon baked apples are a warm and comforting dessert, rich in fiber, antioxidants, and natural sweetness, suitable for those managing insulin resistance.

INGREDIENTS

- ➢ 4 medium apples (such as Granny Smith or Honeycrisp)
- ➢ 1 tablespoon melted coconut oil or butter
- ➢ 1 tablespoon pure maple syrup or honey
- ➢ 1 teaspoon ground cinnamon
- ➢ 1/4 cup chopped nuts (such as walnuts or pecans)
- ➢ Greek yogurt or whipped coconut cream for serving (optional)

PREPARATION INSTRUCTIONS

1. Preheat oven to 375°F (190°C). Lightly grease a baking dish with coconut oil or butter.
2. Core each apple and slice off the top to create a small cavity.
3. In a small bowl, combine melted coconut oil (or butter), maple syrup (or honey), and ground cinnamon.
4. Place apples in the prepared baking dish. Spoon the cinnamon mixture into the cavities of the apples.
5. Bake for 25-30 minutes, or until apples are tender and caramelized.
6. Remove from oven and let cool slightly.
7. Serve warm, optionally topped with chopped nuts and a dollop of Greek yogurt or whipped coconut cream.

NUTRITIONAL VALUE

Calories: 180
Protein: 3g
Carbohydrates: 30g
Fiber: 6g
Fat: 7g

Coconut Chia Seed Smoothie Bowl

Coconut chia seed smoothie bowl is a creamy and satisfying breakfast or dessert option, rich in fiber, healthy fats, and antioxidants, suitable for managing insulin resistance.

INGREDIENTS

- 1/4 cup chia seeds
- 1 cup unsweetened coconut milk
- 1 frozen banana
- 1/2 cup frozen pineapple chunks
- 1 tablespoon unsweetened shredded coconut
- Fresh berries and sliced banana for topping

PREPARATION INSTRUCTIONS

1. In a bowl, combine chia seeds and coconut milk. Stir well and refrigerate for at least 1 hour, or until chia seeds have absorbed the liquid and mixture thickens.
2. In a blender, combine soaked chia seed mixture, frozen banana, and frozen pineapple chunks.
3. Blend until smooth and creamy, scraping down the sides as needed.
4. Pour the smoothie into a bowl.
5. Top with unsweetened shredded coconut, fresh berries, and sliced banana.
6. Serve immediately.

NUTRITIONAL VALUE
Calories: 280
Protein: 6g
Carbohydrates: 40g
Fiber: 12g
Fat: 12g

CONDIMENTS AND STOCKS

Homemade Tomato Sauce

Homemade tomato sauce is a versatile and flavorful condiment, rich in antioxidants and vitamins, suitable for enhancing insulin resistance-friendly meals.

INGREDIENTS

- ➤ 1 can (28 oz) crushed tomatoes
- ➤ 2 tablespoons olive oil
- ➤ 1 onion, finely chopped
- ➤ 2 cloves garlic, minced
- ➤ 1 teaspoon dried oregano
- ➤ 1 teaspoon dried basil
- ➤ Salt and pepper to taste
- ➤ Fresh basil leaves for garnish (optional)

PREPARATION INSTRUCTIONS

1. Heat olive oil in a saucepan over medium heat.
2. Add finely chopped onion and sauté for 3-4 minutes until softened.
3. Add minced garlic, dried oregano, and dried basil. Cook for 1 minute until fragrant.
4. Pour in crushed tomatoes and stir to combine.
5. Season with salt and pepper to taste.
6. Simmer over low heat for 20-30 minutes, stirring occasionally, until sauce thickens.
7. Remove from heat and let cool slightly.
8. Use an immersion blender or transfer to a blender to puree until smooth (optional).
9. Garnish with fresh basil leaves before serving.

NUTRITIONAL VALUE

Calories: 50
Protein: 1g
Carbohydrates: 7g
Fiber: 2g
Fat: 3g

Lemon Herb Dressing

Lemon herb dressing is a zesty and light condiment, perfect for salads or as a marinade for poultry and fish, enriched with vitamin C and essential herbs.

INGREDIENTS

- Juice and zest of 1 lemon
- 3 tablespoons olive oil
- 1 clove garlic, minced
- 1 teaspoon Dijon mustard
- 1 teaspoon honey (optional)
- 1 tablespoon chopped fresh parsley
- 1 tablespoon chopped fresh basil
- Salt and pepper to taste

PREPARATION INSTRUCTIONS

1. In a bowl, whisk together lemon juice, lemon zest, olive oil, minced garlic, Dijon mustard, and honey (if using).
2. Stir in chopped fresh parsley and basil.
3. Season with salt and pepper to taste.
4. Use immediately as a dressing for salads or as a marinade for poultry or fish.

NUTRITIONAL VALUE
Calories: 80
Protein: 0g
Carbohydrates: 2g
Fiber: 0g
Fat: 9g

Homemade Chicken Stock

Homemade chicken stock is a nutritious base for soups, stews, and sauces, packed with collagen, amino acids, and essential nutrients, beneficial for managing insulin resistance.

INGREDIENTS

- ➢ 2 lbs chicken bones (necks, backs, wings)
- ➢ 2 carrots, chopped
- ➢ 2 celery stalks, chopped
- ➢ 1 onion, quartered
- ➢ 2 cloves garlic, smashed
- ➢ 1 bay leaf
- ➢ 1 teaspoon whole peppercorns
- ➢ Water, enough to cover ingredients
- ➢ Salt to taste (optional)

PREPARATION INSTRUCTIONS

1. Place chicken bones, chopped carrots, celery, onion, garlic, bay leaf, and peppercorns in a large stockpot.
2. Add enough water to cover the ingredients by about 2 inches.
3. Bring to a boil over high heat, then reduce heat to low.
4. Simmer, uncovered, for 2-3 hours, skimming any foam that rises to the surface.
5. Remove from heat and let cool slightly.
6. Strain the stock through a fine-mesh sieve into a large bowl or container.
7. Discard solids and season with salt to taste, if desired.
8. Allow stock to cool completely before refrigerating or freezing in portions.

NUTRITIONAL VALUE

Calories: 15
Protein: 2g
Carbohydrates: 1g
Fiber: 0g
Fat: 0g

Basil Pesto Sauce

Basil pesto sauce is a vibrant and aromatic condiment, packed with fresh herbs, garlic, and healthy fats, suitable for enhancing insulin resistance-friendly dishes.

INGREDIENTS

- ➢ 2 cups fresh basil leaves, packed
- ➢ 1/3 cup pine nuts or walnuts
- ➢ 1/2 cup grated Parmesan cheese
- ➢ 2 cloves garlic, minced
- ➢ 1/2 cup olive oil
- ➢ Juice of 1/2 lemon
- ➢ Salt and pepper to taste

PREPARATION INSTRUCTIONS

1. In a food processor, pulse basil leaves, pine nuts or walnuts, Parmesan cheese, and minced garlic until coarsely chopped.
2. With the food processor running, slowly drizzle in olive oil until pesto reaches desired consistency.
3. Add lemon juice, salt, and pepper to taste. Pulse to combine.
4. Use immediately as a sauce for pasta, grilled meats, or as a dip.

NUTRITIONAL VALUE

Calories: 150
Protein: 3g
Carbohydrates: 2g
Fiber: 1g
Fat: 15g

Turmeric Ginger Dressing

Turmeric ginger dressing is a tangy and anti-inflammatory condiment, enriched with antioxidants and beneficial spices, suitable for salads or as a marinade.

INGREDIENTS

- ➢ 1/4 cup olive oil
- ➢ Juice of 1 lemon
- ➢ 1 tablespoon grated fresh ginger
- ➢ 1 teaspoon ground turmeric
- ➢ 1 teaspoon honey (optional)
- ➢ Salt and pepper to taste

PREPARATION INSTRUCTIONS

1. In a bowl, whisk together olive oil, lemon juice, grated fresh ginger, ground turmeric, and honey (if using).
2. Season with salt and pepper to taste.
3. Use immediately as a dressing for salads or as a marinade for vegetables, poultry, or fish.

NUTRITIONAL VALUE

Calories: 120
Protein: 0g
Carbohydrates: 2g
Fiber: 0g
Fat: 14g

CONCLUSION

"The Ultimate Insulin Resistance Diet for Beginners" offers a transformative approach to managing insulin resistance, PCOS, weight loss, and preventing prediabetes. By focusing on nutrient-rich whole foods like vegetables, lean proteins, and healthy fats while minimizing sugars and processed foods, this diet stabilizes blood sugar levels and promotes overall health.

Through balanced meals and regular physical activity, individuals like Maya experience not only weight loss but also increased energy and improved hormonal balance. Embracing this diet isn't just about achieving physical changes; it's about reclaiming control over one's health and well-being.

For those considering adopting this lifestyle, remember: each meal is an opportunity to nourish your body and support its resilience against insulin resistance. Start small, experiment with new recipes, and celebrate every positive change, no matter how small. Your journey towards better health is unique, and every step counts towards a healthier, more vibrant future. As Maya found her strength in this diet, so too can you. Embrace the challenge with determination and optimism—your health journey begins now.

NOTE

WEEKLY MEAL PLANNER

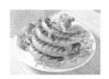 # Weekly Meal Planner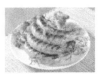

MONDAY
- BREAKFAST
- LUNCH
- DINNER
- SNACK

TUESDAY
- BREAKFAST
- LUNCH
- DINNER
- SNACK

WEDNESDAY
- BREAKFAST
- LUNCH
- DINNER
- SNACK

THURSDAY
- BREAKFAST
- LUNCH
- DINNER
- SNACK

FRIDAY
- BREAKFAST
- LUNCH
- DINNER
- SNACK

SATURDAY
- BREAKFAST
- LUNCH
- DINNER
- SNACK

SUNDAY
- BREAKFAST
- LUNCH
- DINNER
- SNACK

NOTES

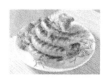 # Weekly Meal Planner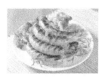

MONDAY
- BREAKFAST
- LUNCH
- DINNER
- SNACK

TUESDAY
- BREAKFAST
- LUNCH
- DINNER
- SNACK

WEDNESDAY
- BREAKFAST
- LUNCH
- DINNER
- SNACK

THURSDAY
- BREAKFAST
- LUNCH
- DINNER
- SNACK

FRIDAY
- BREAKFAST
- LUNCH
- DINNER
- SNACK

SATURDAY
- BREAKFAST
- LUNCH
- DINNER
- SNACK

SUNDAY
- BREAKFAST
- LUNCH
- DINNER
- SNACK

NOTES

Weekly Meal Planner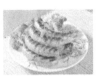

MONDAY
BREAKFAST
LUNCH
DINNER
SNACK

TUESDAY
BREAKFAST
LUNCH
DINNER
SNACK

WEDNESDAY
BREAKFAST
LUNCH
DINNER
SNACK

THURSDAY
BREAKFAST
LUNCH
DINNER
SNACK

FRIDAY
BREAKFAST
LUNCH
DINNER
SNACK

SATURDAY
BREAKFAST
LUNCH
DINNER
SNACK

SUNDAY
BREAKFAST
LUNCH
DINNER
SNACK

NOTES

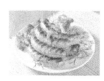 # Weekly Meal Planner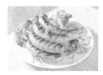

MONDAY
- BREAKFAST
- LUNCH
- DINNER
- SNACK

TUESDAY
- BREAKFAST
- LUNCH
- DINNER
- SNACK

WEDNESDAY
- BREAKFAST
- LUNCH
- DINNER
- SNACK

THURSDAY
- BREAKFAST
- LUNCH
- DINNER
- SNACK

FRIDAY
- BREAKFAST
- LUNCH
- DINNER
- SNACK

SATURDAY
- BREAKFAST
- LUNCH
- DINNER
- SNACK

SUNDAY
- BREAKFAST
- LUNCH
- DINNER
- SNACK

NOTES

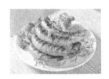 # Weekly Meal Planner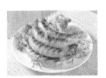

MONDAY
- BREAKFAST
- LUNCH
- DINNER
- SNACK

TUESDAY
- BREAKFAST
- LUNCH
- DINNER
- SNACK

WEDNESDAY
- BREAKFAST
- LUNCH
- DINNER
- SNACK

THURSDAY
- BREAKFAST
- LUNCH
- DINNER
- SNACK

FRIDAY
- BREAKFAST
- LUNCH
- DINNER
- SNACK

SATURDAY
- BREAKFAST
- LUNCH
- DINNER
- SNACK

SUNDAY
- BREAKFAST
- LUNCH
- DINNER
- SNACK

NOTES

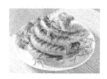 # Weekly Meal Planner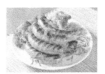

MONDAY
- **BREAKFAST**
- **LUNCH**
- **DINNER**
- **SNACK**

TUESDAY
- **BREAKFAST**
- **LUNCH**
- **DINNER**
- **SNACK**

WEDNESDAY
- **BREAKFAST**
- **LUNCH**
- **DINNER**
- **SNACK**

THURSDAY
- **BREAKFAST**
- **LUNCH**
- **DINNER**
- **SNACK**

FRIDAY
- **BREAKFAST**
- **LUNCH**
- **DINNER**
- **SNACK**

SATURDAY
- **BREAKFAST**
- **LUNCH**
- **DINNER**
- **SNACK**

SUNDAY
- **BREAKFAST**
- **LUNCH**
- **DINNER**
- **SNACK**

NOTES

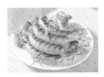 # Weekly Meal Planner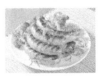

MONDAY
- BREAKFAST
- LUNCH
- DINNER
- SNACK

TUESDAY
- BREAKFAST
- LUNCH
- DINNER
- SNACK

WEDNESDAY
- BREAKFAST
- LUNCH
- DINNER
- SNACK

THURSDAY
- BREAKFAST
- LUNCH
- DINNER
- SNACK

FRIDAY
- BREAKFAST
- LUNCH
- DINNER
- SNACK

SATURDAY
- BREAKFAST
- LUNCH
- DINNER
- SNACK

SUNDAY
- BREAKFAST
- LUNCH
- DINNER
- SNACK

NOTES

Weekly Meal Planner

MONDAY
- BREAKFAST
- LUNCH
- DINNER
- SNACK

TUESDAY
- BREAKFAST
- LUNCH
- DINNER
- SNACK

WEDNESDAY
- BREAKFAST
- LUNCH
- DINNER
- SNACK

THURSDAY
- BREAKFAST
- LUNCH
- DINNER
- SNACK

FRIDAY
- BREAKFAST
- LUNCH
- DINNER
- SNACK

SATURDAY
- BREAKFAST
- LUNCH
- DINNER
- SNACK

SUNDAY
- BREAKFAST
- LUNCH
- DINNER
- SNACK

NOTES

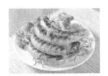 # Weekly Meal Planner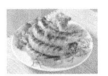

MONDAY

BREAKFAST	
LUNCH	
DINNER	
SNACK	

TUESDAY

BREAKFAST	
LUNCH	
DINNER	
SNACK	

WEDNESDAY

BREAKFAST	
LUNCH	
DINNER	
SNACK	

THURSDAY

BREAKFAST	
LUNCH	
DINNER	
SNACK	

FRIDAY

BREAKFAST	
LUNCH	
DINNER	
SNACK	

SATURDAY

BREAKFAST	
LUNCH	
DINNER	
SNACK	

SUNDAY

BREAKFAST	
LUNCH	
DINNER	
SNACK	

NOTES

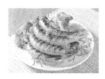 # Weekly Meal Planner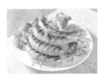

MONDAY
BREAKFAST

LUNCH

DINNER

SNACK

TUESDAY
BREAKFAST

LUNCH

DINNER

SNACK

WEDNESDAY
BREAKFAST

LUNCH

DINNER

SNACK

THURSDAY
BREAKFAST

LUNCH

DINNER

SNACK

FRIDAY
BREAKFAST

LUNCH

DINNER

SNACK

SATURDAY
BREAKFAST

LUNCH

DINNER

SNACK

SUNDAY
BREAKFAST

LUNCH

DINNER

SNACK

NOTES

Thank you for reading the ultimate insulin resistance diet for beginners. We hope these recipes inspire and guide you on your journey to better health and well-being. Your commitment to making positive changes is commendable, and we wish you great success and enjoyment in every meal you create. Please leave a review to help us improve.

Happy cooking!

Made in the USA
Las Vegas, NV
19 September 2024

95514436R00059